THE PREMIER

MCQ FOR POST GRADUATION
UNANI ENTRANCE EXAMINATION

(PREVIOUS EXAMINATION PAPERS OF MD Unani AMU ALIGARH)

THE PREMIER

MCQ FOR POST GRADUATION
UNANI ENTRANCE EXAMINATION

(PREVIOUS EXAMINATION PAPERS OF MD UNANI AMU ALIGARH)

By

Dr. Haqeeq Ahmad
(M.D)
Lecturer, Dept of Ilmul Advia
Hakeem Abdul Hameed Unani Medical College & Hospital,
Dewas, M.P

Dr Izharul Hasan
(M.D)
Lecturer, Dept of Tahaffuzi wa Samaji Tib
Ayurvedic and Unani Tibbia College, Karol Bagh
New Delhi

PREFACE

Students always felt scarcity of quality books in Unani Tib throughout the B.U.M.S student life. This scarcity goes some extra mile when it comes to the study material for the preparation of PG entrance test. While preparing for PG entrance during my students life I found few such books which satisfactorily fulfill the requirement of a students who prepare for entrance test. This problem continued for next generation also, whatever I felt during the preparation. Students used to say that they are not finding good books for entrance test. Then after becoming a lecturer I decided to solve or at least try to solve this problem by writing the books which I fined keeping the problem in mind. The books which I fined beneficial while preparing for PG entrance was the effort of Dr. Ashar Qadeer, Dr. Abdul Bari etc who put the tremendous and some extra ordinary work. In this contest the work of Dr. Ashar Qadeer is worthy to mention here. The wrote different books in the form of MCQs and short notes on different subjects of the Unani Tib I have decided to move their work further forward.

One more important problem which students are facing these days is, they usually study the Unani books and MCQs in Urdu medium and in most PG entrance examinations and Medical Officers examinations, the medium of the questions remains English, although the terms are Unani, this create a confusions in the minds of the students and they are either commit mistakes, resulting in marking wrong answer although they know the correct answer or they leave the questions wondering the negative marking. This ultimately affects the selection after putting lot of hard work.

That's why I decided to solve this problem by writing this book, keeping the medium of the book English, so that while going for entrance test student should not feel some new things all of a sudden and they feel same atmosphere as, while at the time of preparation.

Hope this book will fulfill the requirement of the students preparing for the Ph.D, PG and MO examinations. I have tried at my level best to keep this book free from mistakes but doing mistakes is human nature, so, in this book if there is any mistakes found kindly inform. I will be very thankful and will do the necessary corrections. I will always appreciate the constructive suggestions in the book for the uplift men of the book and Unani Tib as well. The authors would like to receive compliments, comments or criticism from you. We owe a debt of gratitude to all our worthy readers for their overwhelming acceptance and valuable suggestions. Suggestions regarding the subject matter and the pattern shall be welcomed. These may be sent to authors through the publisher or directly via email at dr.haqeeq@gmail.com/drizharnium@gmail.com.

Dr Haqeeq Ahmad
Dr Izharul Hasan

INDEX

1. Usool-e-Tarakeeb ka musanif hai:
a. Najeebuddin Samar Qandi
b. Nafis bin Aoz
c. Zakaria Rhazi
d. Ghulam Jelaani

2. Arq hasil karne ke liye dawa aur paani ka tanasub amooman hota hai:
a. 1 and 20
b. 1 and 15
c. 1 and 10
d. 1 and 16

3. Afshurda ka mafhoom hai:
a. Bahut bareek pisi hoi dawa
b. Usara ka mutradif hai
c. Both a and b
d. None of the above

4. Kushta me istemaal hone wali dhat ki shinakht ke liye istemaal hota hai:
a. Ma-ul-Hayat
b. Ikseer-e-Hayat
c. Both
d. None

5. Hammam Maiya/ Hammam Nariya:
a. Ye Qarrae anbeeq ki ek qism hai
b Isme bilwasta hararat pahuchai jati hai
c. Is ke zariye adwia Mashmooma, phoolo aur phaloo ka khalis arq ya rooh hasil ki jati hai
d. All of the above

6. Shangaraf ko musaffa karte hain:

a. Arqe badiyan me kharal karke

b. Arqe ajwain me kharal karke

c. Arqe gulab me kharal karke

d. Aabe limo me kharal karke

7. Roghan-e-Tila taiyaar kiya jata hai bazariya:

a. Patal Jantar

b. Tareeq-e-Lolbi

c. Garbh Jantar

d. Doli Jantar

8. Zingar bunyadi taur par taiyaar kiya jata hai:

a. Tamba aur sirka ki aamizash se

b. Gandhak aur sammulfaar ki aamizash se

c. Para aur sankhia ki aamizash se

d. Kibreet aur simaab ki aamizash se

9. Amooman jawahiraat aur Hujiriyat kharal kiye jate hain:

a. Sang-e-Siyah me

b. Sang-e-Moosa me

c. Sang-e-Khara me

d. Sang-e-Simaq me

10. One Mishqal equal to:

a. 4.2 gm

b. 3.5 gm

c. 2.5 gm

d. None of the above

11.Jalinoos ke mutabiq Sikta ke mareez ko dafan karne me kitni takhair karni chahiye:

a. 48 hours

b. 24 hours

c. 94 hours

d. 72 hours

12. Zatul janab ghair Haqeeqi ka sabab kiya hai:

a. Ghaleez riyah

b. Waram

c. Sue Mizaj Har

d. Sue Mizaj Barid

13. Urooq ke takkul ke baas nafsuddam aariz hota ho to iska ilaj nihayat duswar hota hai ye kis ka qaul hai:

a. Saikh bu Ali Sina

b. Aristo

c. Jalinoos

d. Buqrat

14. Buqrat ke mutabiq Maus Shaeer kitni khoobiyo ke baas garam marzo me mufeed hai:

a. 15

b. 10

c. 3

d. 11

15. Buqrat ka qaul hai Sar ke dard ka ilaj karna chahiye:

a. Qai se

b. Ishal se

c. Both a and b

d. None of the above

16. Inqalabe Meda ka ilaj karna chahiye:

a. Kasir riyah Advia se

b. Qabiz Advia se

c. Mushil Advia se

d. Lesdar cheezo se

17. Melancholea ki wah qism jisme saudawi khilt dimagh aur us ke urooq me mauzood hain is ka ilaj me mufeed hota hai:

a. Dreedah Afsanteen

b.Matbookh Aftimoon

c. Habbe iyaraj

d. Habbe qauqaiya

18. Dawaon ko ghiza par phailakar kanpati par chispa karne ko kahte hain:

a. Zimad

b. Tila

c. Lazaq

d. Tikoor

19. Barsam ka ilaj kis ke manind karte hai:

a. Sarsam

b. Zatul riya

c. Khafqan

d. Zatul zanab

20. Mushilat ka istemal nahi karna chahiye:

a. Warme masana

b. Warme tihal

c. Warme mirara

d. Warme kabid muhaddab

21. Malencholea ki nabz hoti hai:

a. Sageer, mukhtalif, sulb

b. Azeem mukhtalif layyan

c. Batee,mumtali, mutfawit

d. Sageer zaeef, mutfawit

22. Khoon ki ufoonat se jo bukhar lahiq hota hai aur musalsal chara rahta hai us ko kahte hain:

a. Humme Matbaqa

b. Rabae lazima

c. Rabae daira

d. Humme muhariqa

23. Injeer hamrah akhrot mufeed hai:

a. Hazale kuliya me

b. Zaufe masana me

c. Zaufe kabid me

d. Zaufe qalb me

24. Qurse Tabasheer hamrah Sharbate khashkhash mufeed hai:

a. Hissate masan me

b. Qarooh masana me

c. Warme masana me

d. Silsil boul me

25. Wajaul Fawad kahte hain:

a. Qalb ke Shadeed dard ko

b. Fame Meda ke Shadeed dard ko

c. Gurda ke Shadeed dard ko

d. Aama ke Shadeed dard ko

26. Imsakul Batan mutradif name hai:

a. Qoolinj ka

b. Qabz ka

c. Elaous ka

d. Bawaseer ka

27. Ghusali dast ate hain:

a. Zaufe aama me

b. Zaufe kabid me

c. Zaufe meda me

d. Zaufe gurda me

28. Sara ka mutradif name:

a. Qazoon

b. Kaboos

c. Jamood

d. Kazaz

29. Habbe barhammi mufeed hai:

a. Taqwiyate Dimagh ke liye

b. Tanqia Dimagh ke liye

c. Nazla har ke liye

d. Kaboos ke liye

30. Suda har ka ilaj karna chahiye:

a. Dawae Ghizai se

b. Ghizai dawai

c. Mudirat se

d. Muariqat se

31. Ghib ghair khalis ke liye kiya sahee hai:

a. Madda me balghamiyat hone ki waja se isme sard Advia kam istemaal karni chaiye

b. Mushilat se pahle munzijat hargiz istemaal na karein

c. Khoob muqawwi aur ziyadah miqdar me ghiza de

d. All of the above

32. In simple diffuse goiter there is:

a. Normal T3, T4 And TSH

b. Raised T3, T4 And TSH

c. Raised TSH but normal T3, T4

d. Raised T3 but normal TSH

33. Abrams needle is used for:

a. Bone marrow aspiration

b. Pleural aspiration

c. Accupuncture

d. None of the above

34. The congenital heart disease which is well tolerated upto adult life is:

a. ASD

b. Cyanotic heart disease

c. TOF

d. All of the above

35. Clinical features of Hyperprolactemia is:

a. Galactorrhoea

b. Hypogonadism

c. Both a and b

d. None

36. Prolonged administration of of synthetic glucocoticoids may lead to:

a. Myxoedema

b. Osteogenesis

c. Cushings disease

d. Itrogenic cushings syndrome

37. Bariatric Surgical Procedure is used:

a. To remove foreign body

b. To traet Bulimia nervosa

c. To treat morbid obesity

d. All of the above

38. General features of shocks are:

a. Hypoteension

b. Oligouria

c. Rapid shallow respiration

d. All of the above

39. Loss of sentation of pressure and vibration indicates:

a. Disease of extra pyramidal tract

b. Disease of spinal cord

c. Disease of muscles

d. All of the above

40. Pericardial effusion ki soorat me kis tarah ki pulse milti hai:

a. Pulsus alterans

b. Pulsus Paradoxus

c. Bisferian pulse

d. Delayed pulse

41. Eye ke extraoccular muscles ziyadah tar kis asab se parwarish pate hain:

a. Occulomotor nerve

b. Optic nerve

c. Ophthalmic nerve

d. Trochlear nerve

42. Commonest sign and symtomps of Upper Motor Neuron disease is:

a. Spasticity

b. Numbness

c. Istarkha

d. None of the above

43. Sangdana Murgh ka taaluq tashreehi etibar se kis nizam se hai:

a. NS

b. Digestive system

c. Reproductive system

d. Endocrine system

44. Al-Kunnashul Tabri kis name se famous hai:

a. Moalijate Buqratia

b. Ghanaa Manaa

c. Qarabadeene Aazam wa akmal

d. Qarabadeene Kabir

45. Fad zahar Haiwani hasil hota hai:

a. Bakri se

b. Bandar se

c. Barah singha se

d. All of the above

46. Tiryaqe Pachish ke ajzae tarkeebi me kaun se dawa shamil hai:

a. Haleela zarad

b. Haleela kabli

c. Haleela siyah

d. All of the above

47. Tila Mubahi wa mumsik ka juze khas kiya hai:

a. Post beikh kaneer

b. Post Khashkhash

c. Post Haleela Kabli

d. None of the above

48. Majoon Sarkhas ka istemaal karte hain:

a. Burs me

b. Wajaul mufasil me

c. Suda me

d. Dedane Aama ke ikhraj ke liye

49. Darje zail kaun se dawa Tiryaqe arba ka juz hai:

a. Qurtum

b. Sina makki

c. Habbul Ass

d. Zarawand

50. Majoone zabeeb ka nafa khas hai:

a. Nafae Sara

b. Muqawwi Aazae Raisa

c. Muharike bah

d. Muqawwi Meda

51. Barood ka inventor hai:

a. Hakeem Safyanoos

b. Desqoredos

c. Asqaliboos

d. Jalinoos

52. Amraze saudawi ke ilaj me mustamli hai:

a. Khameera Abresham

b. Khameera khaskhash

c. Majoon Najah

d. Majoon Ushba

53. Fuqaah ka taluq dawa ke kis makhiz se hai:

a. Nabati

b. Haiwani

c. Madani

d. Masnawi

54. Cuscuta reflexa ka maaroof name hai:

a. Kameela

b. Baubarang

c. Aftimoon

d. None of the above

55. Uroos Dar Pardah kis dawa ko kahte hain:

a. Phyllanthus niruri

b. Physalis alkekengi

c. Solanum nigrum

d. Cichorium intybus

56. Darje zail kaun sa fail barge jhao ke sath hai:

a. Taqwiyate Qalb

b. Taqwiyate Meda

c. Taqwiyate Tihal

d. Taqwiyate Gurda

57. Indole alkaloids paye jate hain:

a. Sinkona me

b. Asgandh me

c. Izaraqi me

d. Jozmasal me

58. Kaun se dawa madani nahi hai:

a. Zaitoon bani israil

b. Gile makhtoom

c. Hajruddam

d. Shah pasand

59. Wasmah patte hote hain:

a. Darakht Azlam ke

b. Gainda ke

c. Mughas ke

d. Sanobar ke

60. Darja soam ki dawa hai:
a. Shahitarah
b. Uslusoos
c. Banafsha
d. Kafoor

61. Darje zail me kaun se dawa mafroosh booti hoti hai:
a. Kameela
b. Kaful arnab
c. Zakhm Hyat
d. Kachnal

62. Darje zail me kis ka shumaar baqoolat me hota hai:
a. Khurfa
b. Habbul zalam
c. Habbatul khizra
d. Qaradmana

63. Filfil safaid kis tarah hasil karte hai:
a. Filfil siyah ko multaani mitti me dibokar khusk karke hasil karlete hain
a. Dono alag alag podho se hasil hote hain
c. Filfil siysh ke kachhe fal ko filfil safaid kahte hai
d. Filfil siyah ki oopri kali satah (Epicarp) ko nikal kar hasil karte hain

64. Kitabul asbabul nabat kis ki Tasneef hai:
a. Zakaria Rhazi kki
b. Ishaq bin Hannain

c. Ibne Sina

d. Saufrastus

65. Tanaquz kaifi me do maddao ki ameezash ke bad in me:

a. Haqeeeqi istihala hota hai

b. Haqeeeqi istihal nahi hota hai

c. Dono soortai mumkin hai

d. Advia ki Sabika mahiyat aur soorate nauiya tabdeel ho jati hai

66. Marz ki halat me bamuqabla sehat faqah ko bardasht karne ki salahiyat:

a. Barh jati hai

b. Ghat jati hai

c. Koi faraq nahi parta hai

d. Roz awwal barti hai phir ghati hai

67. Nashif dawa me taseer hoti hai:

a. Mulayyan

b. Kavi

c. Muffateh

d. Jazib

68. Kitabul Taiseer fil mudawat wal Tadabeer ka Musanif kaun hai:

a. Ibne Nadeem

b. Ibne Zohar

c. Ibne Wafid

d. Ibnul Qaf

69. Codiene ka active metabolite hai:

a. Morphine

b. Canrenone

c. Oxazepam

d. Desipramine

70. Mukhashin, musalib, Mukasif, Radae aur Asir taseeraat payi jati hain:

a. Hulu me

b. Afis me

c. Malah me

d. Maseikh me

71. Sibr zard kis qiwam ki dawa hai:

a. Dawae Luzij

b. Dawae Hush

c. Dawae Luabi

d. Dawae Duhni

72. Samandar sokh ka badal hai:

a. Talmakhana

b. Sange busri

c. Samandar phal

d. Sange Sarmahi

73. Risala Yaqooti kis Tabeeb ki Tasneef hai:

a. Ibne Sina

b. Ajmal Khan

c. Ammaduddin

d. Alvi Khan

74. Turbud ke sath Zanjabeel ki ameezash se:
a.Ishal tez ho jate hai
b. Ishal ruk jate hai
c. Ishal kam ho jata hai
d. No effect

75. Anaximenus ne kis unsure ko awwaleen unsure qarar diya:
a. Paani
b. Hawa
c. Aag
d. Mitti

76. Wah Mizaj jo kisi shakhs ke liye us ke jati ahwal ke ziyadah mauzo aur nihayt durust ho aise mizaj ko kiya kahte hai:
a. Mizaj motadil Tibbi Bil Qayas Ilal Dakhil
b. Mizaj motadil Shakhsi Bil Qayas Ilal Kharij
c. Mizaj motadil Shakhsi Bil Qayas Ilal Dakhil
d. Mizaj motadil Tibbi Bil Qayas Ilal Kharij

77. Umr ke darjat me wah kaun sa darja hai jis na aaza barhte hai aur nag hate hai:
a. Sine namu
b. Sine Waqoof
c. Sine kaholat
d. Sine Shaikhokhat

78. Azae raisa aur khidmat ke lihaz se wah khidmat jo kisi rais azu ke fail ke bad waqae ho use kiya kahte hai:
a. Khidmate maudiya kahte hain
b. Khidmate muhayya kahte hain
c. Khidmate uzuiya kahte hain
d. None of the above

79. Kaun se quwwat Tarkeeb wa Tafseel ka kam karti hai:
a. Hisse mushtarak
b. Quwwatw Mutsarfa
c. Quwwate Wahima
d. None

80. Sabse pahle kis Unani Falsafi, Tabeeb ne Unsure Maa ko hi kainat ki paidaish ke silsle me bunyadi juz qarar diya:
a. Hippocrates
b. Galen
c. Thales
d. Aristotle

81. Ghair Tabai balgham ki wah kaunsi qism hai jo sardi khushki ki taraf mail hota hai:
a. Balgham malah
b. Balgham Hamiz
c. Balgham Maseikh
d. Balgham hulu

82. Afal ki ro se faile hazam kis me shumaar kiya jata hai:
a. Afale murakkaba
b. Afale mufarada
c. Afale mushtarakka
d. None of the above

83. Tabeeb mahaz tabiyat ki nigraani ki khidmat anjam deta hai iseliye Tabiyat ka dosra nam rakha gaya:
a. Tabiyat mudabare badan
b. Tabaai
c. Mutbaai
d. None

84. Ghair motadil murakkab me ek sath kitni kaifiateziyadah hoa karti hain:

a. Four kaifiyat
b. Three kaifiyat
c. Six kaifiyat
d. Two kaifiyat

85. Mirra safra kab paida hota hai:

a. Jab raqeeq khoon safra me mil jata hai
b. Jab raqeeq balgham safra me mil jata hai
c. Jab raqeeq safra , balgham me mil jata hai
d. None of the above

86. Quwwate Shoqia ki khadim quwwate kaun se hain:

a. Shahwania aur Ghazbiah
b. Muharika and Mudarika
c. Lamisa and Namia
d. None of the above

87. Mandarja zail me se kin aaza ke taghzia me sauda ka juz shamil nahi hota hai:

a. Tihal
b. Bone
c. Hairs
d. Kabid

88. Waham ka mutradif name kiya hai:

a. Tafakur
b. Takhayul
c. Tadbeer
d. All of the above

89. Decompression sickness is due to:

a. Fat embolism
b. Gas embolism
c. F.B embolism

d. Amniotic embolism

90. Gross infection occurring in Hospital is called:
a. Endogenous infection
b. Exogenous infection
c. Nosocomial infection
d. Itrogenic infection

91. The characteristic features of pus of amoebic liver abscess:
a. Thin blue pus
b. Green colour pus
c. Anchovy sauce pus
d. White colour, bad smell pus

92. Mandarja zail me kaun se alamat, Alamate sudda hai:
a. Jab badan ka rang etidal se ziyadah safaidi mailya zardi mail ho jaye
b. Jab angdai ya jamwahi ki ziyadti ho aur imtalai alamate zahir hon
c. Jab badan me mawad ruk jaye aur rukne ki alamat ke sath tanao ka ehsas ho
d. Both a and b

93. Complications of duodenal ulcer are:
a. Perforation, haemorrhage and obstruction and rarely malignant transformation
b. Perforation, haemorrhage and obstruction and never malignant transformation
c.Only Perforation, haemorrhage and obstruction
d. Both a and b

94. Hyperplasia refers to:
a. Enlargement of the organ or tissue without increase in number of parenchymal cells

b. Enlargement of the organ with increase in number of parenchymal cells

c. Change of one types of cells to another type of cells

d. Disordered cellular development

95. Reehul Shokah kahte hai:
a. Haddi me kisi bairooni sabab se tafaruqe ittesal lahiq hone ko

b. Haddi me kisi andarooni sabab se tafaruqe ittesal lahiq hone ko

c. Aaza ki sakht kea lag alag ho jane ko

d. Taul me tafaruqe ittesal lahiq hone ko

96. Haemolytic anaemia occurs due to:
a. Nuclear maturation defect

b. Unconjugated hyperblirubinaemia

c. Increased red cell obstruction

d. Increased blood loos

97. Wajae Tammadud usd ko kahte hai jis me:
a. Is dard ke sath tanao wa tangi mahsoos ho

b. Is dard ke sath tanao jaisi kaifiat ho

c.Is me yeh ahsas hota hai ki jaise kisi azu ko phara jata hai

d. Is dard me nokai chhuphti haii

98. Diabetic foot is caused due to:
a. Gas Gangrene

b. Dry Gangrene

c. Wet Gangrene

d. Wet Gangrene as well as Gas Gangrene

99. Qoolinj ki halat me Atiba qadam kiya usool murattab kiya hai:
a. Basleeq ki fasad khulwane ki sifarish karte hain

b. Qeefal ki fasad khulwane ki sifarish karte hain

c. Akhal ki fasad khulwane ki sifarish karte hain

d. kisi bhi fasad khulwane se parhaizkarne ki sifarish karte hain

100. Mandarja zail me se kis marz me dalak ki mamno hai:
a. Wajaul asab
b. Farbahi
c. Wajaul urqunnisa
d. Warme Mufasil Haad

101. Hammam Qadmi ka mutradif name hai:
a. Abzan
b. Pashviya
c.Hammam Ramli
d. Hammam Baraqi

102. Ghizae Lateef qaleelul Taghzia ki mishal hai:
a. Zardi Baizae Murgh
b. Maaushaeer
c. Maaul leham
d. Yakhni

103. Hazamat ke fauran bad kis mizaj ke shaks ko aghziae lateefa dene ki ijazat hai:
a. Damwi mizaj
b. Safrawi mizaj
c. Balghami mizaj
d. Saudawi mizaj

104. Khafeef mushily Advia den eke bad kaun se Tadabeer akhtiyar ki izajat hai:
a. Mareez ko sone ki hidayat kare
b. Mareez ko sone na diya jaye
c. Dalak ras ki hidayat kare
d. Riyazat ki hidayat kare

105. Kis wareed ko haftam andam kaha jata hai:

a. Qeefal

b. Abti

c. Akhal

d. Asleem

106. Amale Tamreekh se murad hai:

a. Kisi sayyal dawa ka bazariya huqna badan me dakhil karna

b. Kisi sayyal roghni dawa ka badan par chuprna

c. Kisi sayyal dawa ka bazariya naak me sudakna

d. Kisi sayyal dawa ka bazariya naak me songhna

107. Mouth ke qarooh, Qalaa, Masorhe ke awjaa wa awram, istarkha aur bawaseer lisha me mufeed fasad ki wareed ka name hai:

a. Chhar rag

b. Rag widaj

c. Rag hablul zaraa

d. Rag Qeefal

108. Qasaateri amal istemal me laya jata hai

a. Elaous

b. Ehtabase boul ki halat me

c. Warme masana ki halat me

d. Sue-ul-Qiniya

109. Which one of the following gives nine pairs of posterior intercostals arteries?

a. Descending thoracic aorta

b. Arch of aorta

c. Abdominal aorta

d. Ascending thoracic aorta

110. The perirenal fat is thickest:

a. At the poles

b. Along the borders

c. On the anterior surface
d. On the posterior surface

111. All the following are related to the anterior surface of left kidney except:
a. Spleen
b. Pancreas
c. Duodenum
d. Left Colic flexure

112. Nissel granules are absent in:
a. Dendrites
b. Cell body
c. Nucleus
d. Axon Hillock

113. The common bile duct (in males) is:
a. About 8 cm long and 8 mm in diameter
b. About 7 cm long and 7 mm in diameter
c. About 6 cm long and 6 mm in diameter
d. About 5 cm long and 5 mm in diameter

114. In postero anterior radiograph of the thorax which of the following structure does not from the left margin of heart shadow:
a. Left auricle
b. Pulmonary trunk
c. Arch of aorta
d. SVC

115. What is the length of thoracic part of trachea?
a. 5 cm
b. 7 cm
c. 10 cm
d. 3 cm

116. The spinal cord in the adult, ends inferiorly at the level of:
a. L5 Vertebrae
b. L3 Vertebrae
c. S2-3 Vertebrae
d. L1 Vertebrae

117. A patient is unable to taste a piece of sugar placed on the anterior part of tongue which cranial nerve is likely to have a lesion:
a. Hypoglossal
b. Vagus
c. Facial
d. Glossopharyngeal

118. Which of the following structure can not be palpated by vaginal examination?
a. Sigmoid colon
b. Perineal body
c. Iliopectineal line
d. Ischial spine

119. If the persons diet is composed all most entirely of fat, which of the following condition may occur:
a. Uraemia
b. Ketosis
c. Hyperglycemia
d. None of the above

120. Average quantity of energy liberated per liter of oxygen used in the body is about:
a. 3.825 calories
b. 4.825 calories
c. 5.825 calories
d. 9.424 calories

121. Phosphorylation of glucose to glucose 6- phosphate in liver cells is promoted mainly by:
a. Phophorylase
b. Hexokinase
c. Glucokinase
d. None of the above

122. Optimum Ph for pepsin activity in stomach is:
a. 1to 1.5
b. 1.8 to 3.5
c. 5.8 to 6.5
d. None of the above

123. Beside reflex, effective defication requires:
a. Parasympathetic reflex
b. Sympathetics reflex
c. Local hormones
d. Peritoneointestinal reflex

124. Deficiency of which vitamin causes weakness of collagen fibers:
a. Vitamin A
b. Vitamin B
c. Vitamin C
d. Vitamin D

125. Which of the following is not the result of sympathetic stimulation?
a. Dilated pupil
b. Dilated bronchi
c. Increased peristalsis
d. Contracted pilo erected muscles

126. Emulsification of fats in GIT is caused by:
a. Agitation in stomach
b. Bile salts

c. Lecithin in bile

d. All of the above

127. Vomiting by Chemoreceptor Trigger Zone (CTZ) can be elicited by:

a. Electrical stimulation of the area

b. Morphine

c. Rapidly changing direction of the body

d. All of the above

128. The following about intrinsic factors are correct except:

a. Essential for B12 absorption

b. Secrted by peptic cells

c. Atrophic gastric mucosa leads to its deficiency

d. Is a glycoprotein

129. Coal Tar containing lotions are mainly effective in:

a. Psoriasis

b. Vitiligo

c. Allergics reactions

d. Scabies

130. Acanthosis nigricans is usually:

a. An infective disorder

b. An allergic disorder

c. Associated with obesity

d. None of the following.

131. The difference between Hirsutism and Hypertrichosis is:

a. Hirsutism in females and Hypertrichosis in Males

b. Hirsutism in females and Hypertrichosis in either sex

c. Both condition are same

d. Both condition are seen in either sex

132. Nikolskys sign is seen in:
a. In patient of Pemphigus
b. In patient of Leprosy
c. In patient of Lichen planus
d. In patient of Oral thrush

133. In hair cycle shedding phase is known as:
a. Angen
b. Catagen
c. Telogen
d. Exogen

134. Herpes Zoster ki waja hai:
a. Reactivation of latent Varicella Zoster Virus
b. Recent infection of Varicella Zoster Virus
c. Auto immune disorder
d. Neurological disorder

135. Atopic Dermatitis is classified as:
a. Exogenous Eczema
b. Endogenous Eczema
c. Both
d. None

136. Human Papilloma Virus kis marz ka sabab hai:
a. Qooba
b. Salail
c. Surkh badah
d. Nar farsi

137. Candle green sign kis marz me dekhte hai:
a. Psoriasis
b. Scabies
c. Leucoderma
d. Banatul lail

138. Washam ka matlab hai
a. Jild ke rang ka bigarna
b. Jild par zakhm par jana
c. Jild par godna
d. Jild par bhaddi surkhi paida hona

139. Polio Virus hota hai:
a. RNA Virus
b. DNA Virus
c. ANA Virus
d. PNA Virus

140. Acute respiratory tract infection kis umr ke baccho me mortality ki wajah hai:
a. Below 10 years
b. Below 7 years
c. Below 12 years
d. Below 5 years

141. Sonographic diagnosis of polyhydramnios is made when amniotic fluid index (AFI) is:
a. 5 cm or more
b. 10 cm or more
c. 15 cm or more
d. 20 cm or more

142. Asynclitic engagement is when presenting part is:
a. Occipital parietal
b. Posterior parietal
c. Sagittal suture
d. Anterior parietal

143. Prolactin assay is not indicated in:
a. Oligomenorrhoea
b. Amenorrhea
c. Menorrhagea

d. Delayed puberty

144. Post coital test is done in:
a. Late secretory phase
b. Late proliferative phase
c. Post ovulation
d. None of the above

145. BBT (Basal Body Temperature) increase after ovulation due to increased level of:
a. Oestrogen
b. FSH
c. LH
d. Progesterone

146. Hypomenorrhoea is a condition when the menstrual bleeding:
a. Last for less than 2 days
b. Occurs at interval of 2-3 months
c. Occurs after 35 days
d. None of the above

146. Spinnbarkeit pattern is an indirect evidence of:
a.Proliferative phase
b. Ovulation
c. Secretory phase
d. Anovulation

138. Hasbe zail alamat me se kaun se alamat Marasmus me nahi hoti hai:
a. Gross wastage of muscles
b. Microcephaly
c. Wasting of subcutaneous tissue
d. Marked stunting

149. Baccho me iron deficiency anaemia ki hasbe zail wajohat hoti hai except:
a. Reduced iron intake
b. Decreased iron absorption
c. Increased iron absorption
d. Defective iron metabolism

150. The other name of Cytotrophoblast is:
a. Trophoblastic layer
b. Langhans layer
c. Longitudinal layer
d. None of the above

151. Interstitial Implantation kis din mukamal hota hai:
a. 11th day
b. 21th day
c. 15th day
d. 5th day

152. Daurane hamal, Pre-eclampsia se hasbe zail complications hote hain except:
a. Eclampsia
b. Accidental haemorrhage
c. PPH
d. HELLP Syndrome

153. Spermatogonium se Mature spermatozoa banana me kitna waqt lagta hai:
a. 35 days
b. 61 days
c. 20 days
d. 10 weeks

154. Boorada Aaj mutamil hai:
a. Kasrate haiz me
b. Qaroohe reham me

c. Istaqrare Hamal ke liye
d. Seelanur Reham me

155. Kis ka qaul hai Reham me aliulamoom warme har aur warme sulab hoa karta hai:
a. Allama najeebuddin Samarqandi
b. Seikhur rais Boo Ali Sina
c. Buqrat
d. Galen

156. Piskaeks sign is positive from:
a. 4th week of gestation
b. 5th week of gestation
c. 6th week of gestation
d. 8th week of gestation

157. Signs of bad prognosis of labour are all except:
a. Weak uterine contraction
b. Premature rupture of membrane
c. Full cervical dilation
d. Slow descend of head

158. The hormones produced by fetal testis are:
a. Testosterone
b. DHEA
c. Antimullarian hormone
d. Both a and c

159. The most common cause of Anal fistula is:
a. Tuberculosis
b. Ulcerative colitis
c. Crohns disease
d. Infection of anal glands

160. Death from carcinoma of Penis usually result from:
a. Metastasis of Liver

b. Metastasis of Lung
c. Urinary obstruction
d. Erosion of femoral blood vessels

161. Vericocoele is communal seen on the:
a. Right ankle
b. Left side of scrotum
c. Right side of scrotum
d. Left ankle

162. Curlings ulcers are seen in:
a. Head injury
b. Ulcerative colitis
c. Syphilis
d. Burns

163. Benign prostatic enlagement is due to hyperplasia of:
a. Adenomatous zone
b. Carcinomatous zone
c. Both of the above
d. None of the above

164. Direct Inguinal hernia comes from:
a. Internal inguinal ring
b. Hasselbacks triangle
c. Callots triangle
d. Femoral triangle

165. Erysipelas is caused by:
a. Streptococcus pyogens
b. Streptococcus faecalis
c. Staphylococcus aureus
d. Treponema pallidum

166. Pyogenic liver abscess kis vaja se hota hai:

a. Aspiration
b. Haematogenous
c. Direct contact
d. Lymphatic spread

167. Calcitonin kis type ke cancer ka Tumour marker hai:
a. Anaplastic carcinoma
b. Papillary carcinoma
c. Madullary carcinoma
d. Follicular carcinoma

168. Nipple se khoon ka risna kiya zahir karta hai:
a. Breast abscess
b. Fibroadenoma
c. Duct papilloma
d. Fat necrosis of breast

169. Most common neoplasm of appendix is:
a. Lymphoma'
b. Adenocarcinoma
c. Leiomyosarcoma
d. Argentaffinoma

170. Mandarja zail me se kaun si Pain less, Midline swelling hai:
a.Brachial cyst
b. Thyroglossal cyst
c. Hygroma
d. Carotid body tumour

171. Parotid gland ka sabse common tumour kaun hai:
a. Squamous cell carcinoma
b. Pleomorphic adenoma
c. Adenolymphoma
d. None of the above

172. Which tumour gives frog face deformity?
a. Nasopharyngeal angiofibroma
b. Antrochonal polyp
c. Ethmoidal polyp
d. Nasopharyngeal carcinoma

173. The feature of conductive hearing loss is:
a. Negative Rinnes Test
b. Positive Rinnes Test
c. Webers lateralizes to bed ear
d. More often involve high frequency

174. Abductors of Vocal cord:
a. Cricothyroid
b. Posterior crico artenoids
c. Lateral crico artenoids
d. Thyro artenoids

175. Dissociative anaesthesia is produced by which of the following anaesthetic drugs:
a. Ketamine
b. Thiopentone sodium
c. Midazolam
d. Propofol

176. Which of the following drugs is an example of depolarizing nuscle relaxant?
a. Vecoronium
b. Pancuronium
c. Atracurium
d. Succinyl choline

177. Which of the following anaesthetic techniques is also known as Subarachnoids block:
a. Epidural block

b. Spinal block
c. Caudal block
d. Pudendal block

178. ACYCLOVIR is used in:
a. Bacterial cinjuctivitis
b. Glaucoma
c. Herpes simplex and Herpes Zoster
d. Granulpmatous uveitis

179. Latest treatment of cataract is:
a. Phaco with (Pc) iol
b. Phaco with (A.c) iol
c. Phaco with foldable iol
d. Phaco with multifocal iol

180. When parallel rays of light from infinity come to a focus on the retina, when accommodation is at rest is called:
a. Ametropia
b. Emmetropia
c. Hyper metropia
d. Myopia

181.Wool Sorter Disease ka doosra name kiya hai:
a. Cutaneous anthrax
b. Pulmonary anthrax
c. Intestinal anthrax
d. Renal anthrax

182. Kaun se Tibb Middle of civilization kahlati hai?
a. Roman Mdicine
b. Egyptian Mdicine
c. Greek Mdicine
d. Mesoptamian Mdicine

183. Antigen Shift is seen in:
a. Influenza A
b. Influenza B
c. Influenza C
d. Hepatitis B

184. Mutnawalat mandarja zail teen taur par asar karte hain except:
a. Fail bil kaifiat
b. Fail bil kimiyat
c. Fail bil unsur
d. Fail bil johar

185. Bhopal gas tragedy is an example of:
a. Propagated epidemics
b. Slow epidemics
c. Modern epidemics
d. Point source epidemics

186. Pani badan ki tarkeeb me is tarah shamil hota hai ki:
a. Is ki soorate nauiya badalti hai lekin juze badan nahi hota hai
b. Is ki soorate nauiya badalti hai lekin juze badan hota hai
c. Is ki soorate nauiya badalti badalti nahi aur nahi juze badan hota hai
c. Is ki soorate nauiya badalti nahi hai lekin juze badan banta hai

187. COBRA snake venum is:
a. Neurotoxic
b. Musculotoxic
c. Vasculotoxic
d. Nephrotoxic

188. Two poisons when administered simultaneously may cause toxic symptoms due to:
a. Synergism
b. Toxicity
c. Adverse reaction
d. Similar effects

189. In case of judicial hanging the heart may continue to beat for:
a. 30 minutes
b. 10 minutes
c. 15-20 minutes
d. 40 minutes

190. Pugilistic attitude is due to
a. Coagulation of proteins of muscles
b. Loss of sodium from tht muscles
c. Loss of water from tht muscles
d. Loss of potassium from tht muscles

191. Which of the following is known as Spinal poison?
a. Abrus precatorius
b. Croton tiglium
c. Nicotine
d. Nux vomica

192. Fatal dose of Arsenic in adult is:
a. 10-15 mg
b. 50-75 mg
c. 80-90 mg
d. 120-200 mg

193. Gastric lavage is contraindicated mainly in corrosive poisoning except:
a. Carbolic acid
b. Nitric acid
c. Caustic soda

d. Salicylic acid

194. Gettlers test is done in:
a. Hanging
b. Drowning
c. Strangulation
d. Fire Arm Injury

195. Most reliable methods of identification of an individual is:
a. Dactylography
b. Scars
c. Anthropometry
d. Hand writing

196. Inquest is done in following cases except:
a. Suicide
b. Dowry death in India
c. Death after 24 hours of admission to a hospital
d. Death under anaesthesia

197. Which of the following is not the immediate sign of death?
a. Insensibility and loss of voluntary power
b. Cessation of respiration
c. Cessation of circulation
d. Changes in the eyes

198. The waste water from a community containing solid and liquid excreta called:
a. Sewage
b. Sullage
c. Night soil
d. Refuse

199. The recommended daily requirement of Vitamin A for adult is:
a. 400 Micrograms
b. 500 Micrograms
c. 600 Micrograms
d.900 Micrograms

200. WHO certified the global eradication of Small pox in the year:
a. May 1980
b. May 1970
c. April 1948
d. April 1980

MD AMU ENTRANCE EXAMNATION ANSWERS KEY 2014-15

1. A	2. A	3. B	4. A	5. D
6. D	7. A	8. A	9. D	10. A
11. D	12. A	13. A	14. B	15. A
16. D	17. B	18. C	19. D	20. D
21. A	22. B	23. A	24. B	25. B
26. B	27. B	28. A	29. A	30. B
31. A	32. A	33. B	34. A	35. C
36. D	37. C	38. D	39. B	40. B
41. A	42. A	43. B	44. A	45. D
46. A	47. A	48. D	49. D	50. A
51. A	52. D	53. A	54. C	55. B
56. C	57. C	58. D	59. A	60. D
61. C	62. A	63. D	64. D	65. B
66. A	67. D	68. B	69. A	70. B
71. B	72. A	73. C	74. A	75. B
76. C	77. B	78. A	79. B	80. C
81. B	82. B	83. B	84. D	85. B
86. A	87. D	88. B	89. B	90. C
91. C	92. B	93. B	94. B	95. B

96. B 97. B 98. C 99. D 100. D
101. B 102. B 103. B 104. B 105. C
106. B 107. A 108. B 109. A 110. B
111. C 112. D 113. A 114. D 115. A
116. D 117. C 118. C 119. B 120. B
121. C 122. B 123. A 124. C 125. C
126. D 127. D 128. B 129. A 130. C
131. B 132. A 133. D 134. A 135. B
136. B 137. A 138. C 139. A 140. D
141. D 142. D 143. C 144. B 145. D
146. A 147. B 148. B 149. C 150. B
151.A 152.C 153.B 154.C 155.A
156.D 157.C   158.D 159.D 160.D
161.B 162.D 163.A 164.B 165.A
166.B 167.C 168.C 169.B 170. B
171.B 172.A 173.A 174.B 175. A
176.D 177.B 178.C 179.D 180. B
181.B 182.D 183.A   184.B 185. D
186.C 187.A 188.A 189.C 190. A
191.D 192.D 193.A 194.B 195. A
196.C 197.B 198.A 199.C 200. A

1. Kashrate attas ki soorat me
a. Dimagh ka tanqia karai
b. Dimagh me tabreed wa taskeen paida kare
c. Muqwwi dimagh Advia istemal karai
d. Imala ki garz se pashwia karai

2. Bawasir shiftah ka hota hai:
a. Urooq ka sudda
b. Khooni jala hoa madda
c. Safarawi jala hoa madda
d. Chhot ka lagna

3. Marz sil la ilaz hai
a. Sheikh ke nazdeek
b. Razi ke nazdeek
c. Jalinoos ke nazdeek
d. Buqrat ke nazdeek

4. Humme istifraghiah ka taluque kis jins se hai:
a. Humm-e-Yaum
b. Humm-e-Diqqi
c. Humm-e-Khilti
d. All of the above

5. Siddat dard ke baas baz auqat mareez khukashi ke irtikaab ke liye ammadah ho jata hai:
a. Suda shaqiqa me
b. Suda baize khozah me
c. Suda usaba me
d. Suda bukhari me

6. Sar ke posterior part me dard hota hai:
a. Suda haar sada me

b. Suda barid sada me

c. Suda haar maddi me

d. Suda barid maddi me

7. Zaghot ka mutradif naam kiya hai:

a. Mania

b. Melancholea

c. Kaboos

d. Sarsam maraqi

8. Faranitus kahte hai:

a. Suda damwi ko

b. Suda safarawi ko

c. Sarsam damwi ko

d. Sarsam safrawi ko

9. Marz bavaiyaten ka taluque kis marz se hai:

a. Kuliya se

b. Masana se

c. Eye se

d. Ear se

10. Zaghtul qalb ka taluque kis khilt se hai:

a. Khilte dam

b. Khilte safara

c. Khilte sauda

d. khilte bagham

11. Mndarza zail me kaun sa sabab istarkha ka nahi hai:

a. Dafae bohrani

b. Inkhalai mufasal

c. Sue mizaj

d. Balghame basoor

12. Jab tihal barh jata hai to jism lagar ho jata hai aur jab tihal lager ho to jism moota ho jata hai kis ka qaul hai:
a. Booali sina ka
b. Jalinoos ka
c. Buqrat ka
d. Zakaria Razi ka

13. Imtlai Riya me kaun se fasad ka kholna mufeed hai:
a. Akhal
b. Basleeq
c. Both a & b
d. None of the above

14. Ibtidai marz me Huqna karana kis me mufeed hai:
a. Jamoodul sadar
b. Nafshul midda
c. Qeemul sadar
d. None of the above

15. Glasgow coma scale me Spontaneous eye opening score hota hai:
a. 3
b. 4
c. 0
d. 1

16. Recurrent pneumonia at the same site or pneumonia slow responding to treatment suggest the possibility of:
a. Bronchial carcinoma
b. Bronchiactesis
c. Pulmonary tuberculosis
d. Lung abscess

17. When breathlessness is the dominant features of myocardial ischemia it is known as:

a. Angina equivalent

b. Angina pectoris

c. Orthopnea

d. All of the above

18. Boul-e-Aswad kis marz par dalalat karta hai:

a. Shiddat-e ahraq

b. Zehar khuraani

c. Hazal-e-Kuliya me

d. None of the above

19. Boul-e-Ghisali milta hai:

a. Sue mizaj meda me

b. Qarooh-e-Masana

c. Hazal-e-Kuliya me

d. None of the above

20. Humm-e-Mevi me nabz milti hai:

a. Saree mumtali layyun wa matraqi

b. Mutwatir wa zaeef

c. Mutwatir wa sulb

d. All of the above

21. Humm-e- Sonukhus ki nabz hoti hai:

a. Saghir wa zaeef sulb

b. Saghir wa zaeef wa layyun

c. Saree wa sulb

d. Azim wa quwwa wa saree wa mutwatir wa mumtali

22. Bakhrul anaf me mufeed hai:

a. Aabe anaar ko naak me tapkana

b. Aabe Kasni ko naak me tapkana

c. Saad kofi pani me pess kar naak me tapkana

d. Aabe Moli ko naak me tapkana

23. Taqalub nafas kahte hai:
a. Us matli ko jo lazim aur deer pa ho
b. Zauf ishtiha ko
c. Zauf hazam ko
d. Kashrate ishtiha ko

24. Ananat me:
a. Mareez wazeefa tanasuli par bilkul qadir nahi hota hai
b. Azae tanasul me kamil intishar nahi hota hai
c. Waqt se pahle injal ho jata hai
d. Ehtalam bilkul nahi hota hai

25. Intalaq-e-badan se murad hai:
a. Meda ke andaroono tabqa me zakham ho jata hai
b. Haiza
c. Jighar ke ishal
d. Ishal dauri

26. Nuskha khalal shikam hai:
a. Barg gaozaban, badiyan, unnab, sapistan bahidana
b. Barg gaozaban, badiyan, ghule banafsha maveez munaqa, bekh kasni
c. Badiyan, Uslussoos, ersa, ustokhuddos, Kasni
d. Unnab, tukhm khatmi, maveez munaqa , ghule bafsha, unnab, sapistan

27. Humme muhariqa jins hai:
a. Humm-e-Damwi ki
b. Humm-e-Gib ki
c. Humm-e-Balghami ki
d. Humm-e-Saudawi ki

28. Kaboos paish khema hai:
a. Sara ka
b. Melancholia
c. Sarsam ka

d. Falij ka

29. Sarsam ke mawad ke liye imala ka bahtareen zarai hai:
a. Ishal
b. Talyyun
c. Fasad
d. Passena

30. Aksar aqsam nazla me mufeed hai:
a. Hubbe shifa
b. Qurse dawushifa
c. Hubbe karanjawa
d. Hubbe jawahar

31. Gurdah me pathri banana ke two asbab hain ghaliz maddah ghaliz maddah ka rukna, kis ka qaul hai:
a. Jalinoos
b. Buqrat
c. Boo ali Sina
d. Zakaria Razi

32. Kia azu ke amraz me quwwa mudirat ka istemal mamno hai:
a. Amraz-e-Masana
b. Amraz-e-Gurdah
c. Amraz-e-Halbain
d. Amraz-e-Jigar

33. Qaroora me sakht badbo ka hona kis par dalalat karta hai:
a. Safra
b. Sauda
c. Balgham
d. Dam

34. Humm-e-Yaum warmia me nabz hoti hai:
a. Sagir, bate aur mutfavit
b. Azim saree aur mutfavit
c. Azim saree aur mutvatir
d. Sagir zaeef aur bate

35. Nettle rash is known in Unani Medicine as:
a. Jarab
b. Hikkah
c. Shara
d. Basoorat

36. Balon ki sufaid hone ki wajah takaruj hai yeh qaul kis ka hai:
a. Razi
b. Jalinoos
c. Sheikh
d. Buqrat

37. Hafiz-e-Shar Advia wah hain jin ke ander:
a. Lateef hararat ho
b. Quwwate jazba ho
c. Quwwate qabiza ho
d. All of the above

38. Which gland is responsible for immunity?
a. Thyroid gland
b. Pancreas gland
c. Thymus gland
d. Pituitary gland

39. A patient of maculopapular rashes, itching mostly in night's gives history of whole family involvement of similar condition..........your diagnosis will be:
a. Urticaria
b. Impetigo
c. Scabies

d. Herpes Simplex

40. Kulf me bairooni taur par mustamil dawa hai:
a. Baqlah
b. Babchi
c. Beikh badiyan
d. Asgand

41. Amraz-e-jild ke ilaj me leech ka istemal nihait mufeed hai yeh kis tabeeb ka qaul hai:
a. Jalinoos
b. Buqrat
c. Raban Tabri
d. Seikh Ibne sina

42. Sankhia aur para ke murakkabat mufeed hain:
a. Syphilis
b. Ringworm
c. Gastritis
d. Jaul baqar

43. Allergy ki soorat me mediators ho sakte hai
a. Acetylcholine
b. Leukotrienes
c. Protacyclin
d. None of the above

44. Tricology me kis ke bare me study karte hai:
a. Borho ke amraz me
b. Purane amraz me
c. Amrze khabisha
d. Amraze shaar

45. Dalak istedad kab ki jati hai:
a. Before exercise
b. After exercise

c. In empty stomach
d. None of the above

46. Mandarza zail me kaun se dawa mana e arq hai:
a. Dhatora
b. Khaksi
c. Tukhm Saljam
d. None of the above

47. Siddain ke zerei hisse me hajamat bil shurt kiis marz me karte hai:
a. Amenorrhea
b. Kasrate tamas
c. Usre tamas
d. Uqr

48. Kemoosh ke aetibar se Maullaham, Yakhni aur zardi baizah murg neem barast hain:
a. Ghiza-e-Lateef kaseerul Taghzia jaiyadul kemoos
b. Ghiza-e-Lateef kaseerul Taghzia raddiul kemoos
c. Ghiza-e-Lateef qaleelul Taghzia jaiyadul kemoos
d. Ghiza-e-Lateef qaleelul Taghzia raddiul kemoos

49. Jild ko needles ke zariyae god kar bareek shighaf bana kar dawa pahuchana kiya kahlata hai:
a. Amal-e- Talqeeh
b. Amal-e- Tateeh
c. Amal-e- Kai
d. Hazamat

50. Imtilah bahasbul aoviah ki tadbeer ilaj hai:
a. Hammam
b. Fasad
c. Riyazat
d. Taareeque

51. Kaun se tadbeer mudirat-e-Amal ko quwwa karti hai:

a. Tabreed jild

b. Pashviyah

c. Inkabab

d. Bakhoor

52. Kisi uzue me kashrate mavad ki soorat me munasib tadbeer ilaj kiya hai:

a. First Fasad then Hajamat

b. First Hajamat then Fasad

c. First Dalak then Hajamat

d. First Mhajama nari then Hajamat

53. Marz muhhaiyaj kahte hai:

a. Jis marz me nuzaj ke intezar ke baghair istifragh dena jaiz ho

b. That amarz jin me nuzaj ke baad istifragh dena jaiz ho

c. Amraz-e-Haadatul muzminat

d. None of the above

54. Mushil dawa khane ke baad sona mushil ke amal ko:

a. Quwwa karta hai

b. Zaeef karta hai

c. Koi asar zahir nahi hota hai

d. Har mizaj ke askhas me alag alag asarat jahir hote hai

55. Badam talakh ki talkhi kis madda waja se hoti hai:

a. Fatty acid

b. Hydrocyanic acid

c. Fixed oil

d. Tannic acid

56. Bareek peesna kis istilah ka mafhoom hai:
a. Tamreekh
b. Tasveel
c. Salaiyah
d. Aqad

57. Usool-e-Dawa sazi par mushtamil Kitab Risalh fi tarkeebul advia kis musanif ki hai:
a. Najeebuddin Samarqandi
b. Daud bin abu lubyaan
c. Ibn-e-Jazar
d. Abul abbas

58. What is the first line treatment for long term control of bronchial asthma?
a. Inhaled corticosteroid
b. Theophylline
c. Salbutamol
d. Oral prednisoline

59. Which of the following are most likely to produce hypoglycemia?
a. Metformin
B. Sulphonylureas (Glibenclamide etc.)
c. Glucagon
d. Corticosteroids

60. Which of the following is diagnostic for opium/Morphine Poisoning?
a. Loss of planter reflex
b. Dilated pupil
c. Pinpoint pupil
d. Facial edema

61. Which of the following precaution is needed in therapy with aminophylline?
a. Oral administration only
b. Slow IV Injection/Infusion
c. Rapid IV Injection
d. Administration of empty stomach

62. The study of the biochemical and physiological effects of drugs and their mechanism of action is called:
a. Pharmacoepidemiology
b. Pharmacokinetics
c. Pharmacodynamics
d. Toxicology

63. Mulatifat me tukhm Turb ki aamezash ki kiya wajah hai:
a. Sareeun nafooz banana
b. Baeeun nafooz banana
c. Talkhi ko door karna
d. Qai auar tasheer ko kam karna

64. Hamiz ajza par mushtamil dawaain kis fail ki hamil hoti hai:
a. Musakhin
b. Murkhi
c. Haliq
d. Zajib

65. Iyaraj loghazia ka juz-e-Khas kiya hai:
a. Turbud
b. Kharbaq
c. Sibr
d. Jalapa

66. Qurs-e-Kafoor me zafran ki shamooliyat ki wajah hai:

a. Izafa quwwat

b. Taqleel-e-Mikdare khurak

c. Badarqiyat

d. Hasasiyat ko kam karna

67. Darje zail Advia me dastaavar dawa ki shinakht kijiye:

a. Abhal

b. Shaum

c. Sumaq

d. Narmushk

68. Risala Atrilal ke musanif ka naam hai:

a. Meer mohammad husaiin sherazi

b. Imadduddin sheerazi

c. Ibne baitar

d. Hakeem Jullur-Rehman

69. Which of the following drug is kishtinuma?

a. Aspaghol

b. Hathi sondhi

c. Halha jorhi

d. Kafgair

70. Mizanuttib kis ki tasneef hai:

a. Akbar arzani

b. Mohammad husain sherazi

c. Imadduddin sheerazi

d. Azam khan

71. Rishalah nabeez ke musanif ka naam hai:

a. Qutabin Lauqa

b. Jorjas

c. Rofas

d. Jalinoos

72. Mughash kis dawa ka mutradif hai:

a. Meda lakdi

b. Kaifal

c. Amla

d. Malkangni

73. Neelofar ka mashoor naam hai:

a. Padmani

b. Tajqalmi

c. Falsah

d. Jalapa

74. Habb-e-Zeeqan nafas ka main ingredient kiya hai:

a. Qaranuail

b. Kakra Singi

c. Uslusoos

d. Arosa

75. Darje zail murakkabat me se kis murakkab ka main ingredient Aabresham hai:

a. Mufareh barid

b. Mufareh Saikhur raish

c. Mufareh motadil

d. All of the above

76. Kharchang ka mutradif naam kiya hai:

a. Barahsingha

b. Satraaerabi

c. Sadaf kharmohra

d. Kekra

77. Darje zail kis murakkab me luk shamil hai:

a. Safoof mohzal

b. Majoon dabidulwarad

c. Both a and b

d. None of the above

78. Kaun se dawa muzafe qalb tasheer rakhti hai
a. Kutki
b. Shailam
c. Beesh
d. All of the above

79. Zarareeh kis fail ki hamil hoti hai
a. Mughri
b. Muqawwi qalb
c. Mudir boul
d. Manai hamizat

80. Kaun se dawa nasif hai:
a. Khatmi
b. Aspaghol
c. Tabasheer
d. Kuchla

81. Jamadat hote hai:
a. Mantaraq
b. Ghair mantaraq
c. Both a and b
d. None of the above

82. Fateela ka istemaal kiya jata hai:
a. Eye and ear
b. Maqad
c. Reham
d. All of theabove

83. Kushta musalas mufeed hita hai:
a. Surate injal mw
b. Saqoote qalb me
c. Hissate kuliya
d. None of the above

84. Kameela kiya hai?
a. Oleo-Gum
b. Gum
c. Dried pulp of a fruit
d. None of the above

85. Kaun sa yashab bahtar shumaar kiya jata hai?
a. Kafoori
b. Sabz
c. Sabz zardi mail
d. Sabz sufaidi mail

86. Ahraque Aqrab Ke liye amooman nar bichho ka istemal karte hain jis ki sinakht hai ki wah:
a. Tawana aur afal hota hai
b. Lagar aur ghair fual hota hai
c. Neesh ka rang banafsi hota hai
d. None of the above

87. Biryan ka amal kiya jata hai:
a. Tootia sabz par
b. Sartan
c. Amaltas par
d. Sankhia par

88. Saiyaf me istemal kiya ja sakta hai:
a. Jalateen
b. Glycerin
c. Water
d. None of the above

89. Bakhtaj ke liye kaun se maroof istalah istemal ki jati hai:
a. Joshandah
b. Khesandah

c. Julal

d. Sheerah

90. Jab haboob ka inhazam meda ke bajay intestine me karana maqsad ho to kiya jata hai:
a. Ghulaf-e- halami
b. Ghulaf-e- Shakar
b. Ghulaf-e-Nuqra
c. Ghulaf-e- Qarni

91. Sharbat ka qiwam maloom karne ke liye jo aala istemal kiya jata hai use kahte hai:
a. Refracto meter
b. Muffle furnace
c. Hydrometer
d. Barometer

92. Ma-us-Shaeer mohamis taiyar kiya jata hai:
a. Chhane ko mohamis kar ke
b. Jao ko bhoon kar ke
c. Wheat ko bhoon kar
d. All of the above

93. Bahut baareek safoof kise kahte hai?
a. Aesa safoof jo chhalni no. 355 se guzar jai
b. Aesa safoof jo chhalni no. 250 se guzar jai
c. Aesa safoof jo chhalni no. 125 se guzar jai
d. None of the above

94. Qarabadeen-e-Kabir ka musanif kaun hai:
a. Hakeem kabiruddin
b. Hakeem Akbar arzani
c. Hakeem mohammad Hussain Khan
d. Hakeem Abdul Lateef Fasafi

95. Darje zail me kaun se shaqal Muhaal hai?

a. Arqe Sammulfar

b. Roghane Sammulfar

c. Johare Sammulfar

d. None of the above

96. Mahloob aur dhanab ki istelah mustamil hai:

a. Para ki tasfia ke liye

b. Abrak ki tasfia ke liye

c. Khrateen ki tasfia ke liye

d. All of the above

97. Cloudy swelling commonly found in:

a. Heart

b. Liver

c. Kidney

d. All of the above

98. Warm-e-Falghamooni ka sabab hai:

a. Khoon

b. Balgham

c. Safra

d. Sauda

99. The common cause of acute pancreatitis is:

a. Cholelithiasis

b. Alcoholism

c. Cholelithiasis & Alcoholism

d. Only cholelithiasis

100. Which is a DNA virus?

a. Hepatitis A virus

b. Hepatitis B virus

c. Hepatitis C virus

d. All of the above

101. Which of the following is true statement for curling ulcer?
a. It is type of stress ulceration of stomach and duodenum
b. It is an ulcer produced by a result of pressure necrosis
c. It is a type of mouth ulceration
d. External ulcers on body surface as a result of burn

102. Which of the following is true for the condition of metabolic acidosis?
a. The respiration rate and depth of respiration are increased
b. The respiration rate and depth of respiration are decreased
c. Its leads to bradycardia
d. No change occur in the rate and depth of respiration

103. Tongue ke carcinoma ki sab se ziyadah common site kaun se hai:
a. Tip
b. Lateral margin
c. Base
d. Root

104. Proximal ulna fracture and radial head ke dislocation ko:
a. Monteggia fracture kahte hai
b. Coles fracture kahte hai
c. Galezzi fracture kahte hai
d. None of the above

105. Islamic period ka kaun Jarrah alate jarahi ka mojid kahlata hai:
a. Zakaria Razi
b. Abu Ali Ibn-e-Sina
c. Ibn-e- Zohar
d. Abul Qasim Zohravi

106. Fracture of Humerus me kis asab ke majroh hone ke imkanat hai:
a. Median
b. Ulnar
c. Radial
d. Axillary

107. What is the most appropriate method for diagnosis of early carcinoma of mid oesophagus?
a. X-Ray chest PA view
b. Bronchoscopy
c. Barium meal and fallow through
d. Upper G.I Endoscopy

108. Perthes test kis marz ke ilaj me istemal hota hai:
a. Burgers disease
b. Varicose of veins
c. Reynaud's disease
d. None of the above

109. The central transparency is maintained by
a. Keratocytes
b. Bowman's membrane
c. Descents membrane
d. Endothelium

110. The posterior urethra is best visualized by:
a. Static cytogram
b. Retrograde Urethrogram
c. Voiding cytogram
d. CT cystogram

111. The palatine tonsil receives its arterial supply from all of the following except:
a. Facial
b. Ascending palatine
c. Sphenopalatine
d. Dorsal lingual

112. Which of the following best represents Ranula?
a. A type of epulis
b. Thyroglossal cyst
c. Cystic swelling in the floor of mouth
d. Forked Uvula

113. One 13 years old boy with sudden onset of scrotal pain. On examination the testis is enlarged and tender, which of the following is the most appropriate management:
a. Immediate exploration
b. Antibiotics
c. Psychiatric evaluation
d. Only analgesics

114. During surgery of Hernia, the sac of strangulated inguinal hernia should be open at the:
a. Neck
b. Body
c. Fundus
d. At deep ring

115. The treatment of choice for mucocoele of gall bladder is:
a. Aspiration of mucus
b. Cholecystectomy
c. Cholecystostomy
d. Antibiotic and observation

116. The diagnosis of congenital mega colon is confirmed by:
a. Clinical features
b. Barium enema
c. Rectal biopsy
d. Rectosigmoidoscopy

117. Nitrous oxide is:
a. A potent analgesics but a weak anesthetic agent
b. A very effective and a potent anesthetic agent but weak analgesics
c. A weak anesthetic agent and a very weak analgesic agent
d. A weak analgesic agent and a weak anesthetic agent

118. Which of the following is a depolarizing muscle relaxant?
a. Pancuronium
b. Suxamethonium
c. Vecuronium
d. Atracurium

119. Which of the following is not a muscle relaxant?
a. Neostigmine
b. Scoline
c. Pavulon
d. Norcuron

120. Local anesthetic agent drug is injected in subarachnoid space in?
a. Epidural anaesthesia
b. Caudal shock
c. Spinal anaesthesia
d. All of the above

121. Accidental Dural puncture is complication of?
a. Spinal anaesthesia

b. Epidural anaesthesia
c. Brachial plexus block
d. All of the above

122. Ketamine is contraindication of?
a. Shock
b. Children
c. Minor surgical procedure
d. All of the above

123. Which of the following is a non depolarizing muscle relaxant?
a. Suxamethonium
b. Atracurium
c. Propofol
d. Ether

124. Mashoor and maroof fasafi aflatoon(Plato) ke sagirdon me sab se jaleelur qadr falsafi wa Tabeeb kaun guzra hai:
a. Suqraat
b. Jalinoos
c. Arastu
d. None of the above

125. Arabic zubaan me likhi jane wali fane tib ki first book kaun se hai:
a. Firdosul hikmat
b. Alqanoon fit Tib
c. Kitabul tib alarab
d. None of the above

126. Ibn-e-Sina ka zamana hayat kab se kab tak ka hai:
a. 960-1037AD
b. 890-937AD
c. 1070-1160 AD

d. None of the above

127. Tezaab-e-shorah (Nitric acid), Tezaab-e-Gandhak (Sulphuric acid) kis kemiyahdah Tabeeb ki ejad hain:
a. Ibne Nafis
b. Ibne baitar
c. Ibne juzl
d. Jabir bin Hayan

128. Us Tabeeb ka naam batai jo 1126 AD me Qurtabah (cordova) me paida hoa aur kitabul kuliyat name mashoor tasneef ka khaliq hai:
a. Ibne Zohar
b. Ibne Rushd
c. Ibne juzla
d. Ibne baitar

129. Quwwat-e-Tabaiyah ki taqseem awal kiya hai:
a. Hafiza wa basira
b. Hasia wa murakkabah
c. Ghazia wa namia
d. Masika wa dafia

130. Quwwate hawania me quwwate munfaila kiya fail anjam deti hai:
a. Dauran-e-Khoon
b. inqabaz wa inbasat qalb ka
c. Infalate nafsania
d. None of the above

131. Asbab-e-Soriyah ki nishandahi kijiye:
a. Mizaj wa quwwa
b. Arwah wa quwwa
c. Mizaj wa arwah
d. All of the above

132. Aaza ke aetibar se qism fauqul quwwa ka kiya mizaj hai:
a. Har ratab
b. Barid ratab
c. Har yabis
d. Barid yabis

133. Agar kisi shaks ki harkat doodiya tez aur B.P kam ho to us ka mizaj kiya honga:
a. Har ratab
b. Har yabis
c. Barid ratab
d. Barid yabis

134. Mandarja zaik me sharait taghzia kiya hain:
a. Mutwazan ghiza ka lena
b. Kaifiyat ke aetibar se ghiza ka accha hona
c. Kaifiyat me ghiza aur badan ka motadil hona
d. None of the above

135. Ahal-e-hind ka mizaj kis jins ke tahat bayan kiya jayega:
a. Mizaj motadil tibbi naui kharji
b. Mizaj motadil tibbi sanfi kharji
c. Mizaj motadil tibbi sanfi dakhli
d. None of the above

136. Aqleem chharam ko aqleem panjam par joi fauqiyat hasil nahi hai yeh kis ka statement hai:
a. Raban Tabri
b. Abu bakar Zakaria Rhazi
c. Ibne Rushd
d. Ali ibne abbas majosi

137. Sine nammu ke kitne darjat hote hain:
a. 4
b. 5

c. 3

d. None of the above

138. The following statement about the vertebral artery is correct except that:

a. It is a branch of first part of subclavian artery

b. It passes through the foramen transversarum to reach the cranial cavity

c. It anastomoses with the branch of internal carotid artery

d. It unite to form vertebral artery at lower border of pons

139. About the cranial nerves the following statements are true except:

a. 1, 2 and 8 are sensory

b. 3, 4, 6 and 12 are motor

c. 5, 6, 9. 10 and 11 are mixed

d. All are bilaterally represented in the cortex

140. The parotid gland is supplied by the following nerve:

a. Facial nerve

b. Glossophatyngeal nerve

c. Mandibular nerve

d. Vagus nerve

141. The following are the branches of basilar artery except:

a . Pontine arteries

b. Anterior inferior cerebellar artery

c. Posterior inferior cerebellar artery

d. Superior cerebellar artery

142. The oculomotor nerve supplies the following muscles except:

a. Levator palpabrae superioris

b. Inferior oblique

c. Ciliaris muscle
d. Lateral rectus

143. About the mid brain it is true except:
a. It contain 3rd and 4th cranial nuclei
b. Tumour or hemorrhage may cause hydrocephalus, due to blockage of C. aqueduct
c. It connect the mid brain with the fore brain
d. Tumour or hemorrhage may cause paralysis of muscle of mastication

144. The following muscle is supplied by Radial nerve except:
a. Triceps
b. Teres minor
c. Brachioradialis
d. Extensor carpi radialis longus

145. The following statements regarding heart are correct except that:
a. It supplied by coronary arteries
b. It is covered by double layered pericardium
c. 4 pulmonary veins open in to upper left chamber
d. The anterior cardiac veins opens in to upper left chamber

146. Concerning the subclavian artery the following statement is correct except that:
a. It is the principal artery of head and neck
b. It arises from arch of aorta on left side
c. It continues as axilliary artery at lower border of first rib
d. It is divided into three parts by scalenus anterior

147. The trachea is divided in to two principal bronchi at the level of:
a. L1
b. L4
c. T1

d.T4

148. Shock ka compensated stage kiya hota hai:
a. Non progressive
b. Progressive
c. Irreversible
d. All of the above

149. Cortisol ke Taluque se kiya sahi hai:
a. Stimulates gluconeogenesis
b. Suppress immune system
c. Prevent inflammation
d. All of the above

150. E.C.G me depolarization par point J kaun sa hota hai:
a. When this wave spread on the whole of the heart
b. Jab yeh wave shurooh hoti hai
c. Jab yeh wave, A.V node par pahunchti hai
d. QRS complex ke highest point par

151. Bile salts ka precursor hai:
a. Triglycerides
b. Phospholipids
c. Cholestrol
d. All of the above

152. Saliva secretion is mainly controlled by:
a. Parasympathetic nervous system
b. Sympathetic nervous system
c. Both a & b
d. None of the above

153. Insulin farogh deta hai:
a. Protein synthesis
b. Gluconeogenesis

c. Fat utilization

d. None of the above

154. Tabai jismani hararat me kitne digree izafa par khuliyat barbad hona shurooh ho jate hai:

a. 5^0 F

b. 7^0F

c. 9^0 F

d. 11^0 F

155. Qalb ke do khano (chambers) se khoon shiryain me pahuchta hai:

a. Right atrium & Right ventricle

b. Left atrium & Left ventricle

c. Right ventricle & Left ventricle

d. Right atrium & Left ventricle

156. Sabse jiyadah volume hota hai:

a. Tidal volume

b. Inspiratory reserve volume

c. Expiratory reserve volume

d. Residual volume

157. Embryo me RBCs ki paidaiish sabse pahle kis uzu me hoti hai:

a. Yolk sac

b. Liver

c. Spleen

d. Bone marrow

158. Neonatal Tetanus commonly occurs in:

a. 2-3 days after birth

b. 5-15 days after birth

c. 16-20 days after birth

d. Just after birth

159. All are indicated for whooping cough except:

a. Kakra singhi

b. Lobaan

c. Roghan-e-Kunjad

d. Tukhme baaqla

160. In which of the following disease live vaccine BCG is used:

a. Hepatitis

b. Diphtheria

c. Tuberculosis

d. None

161. Aam taur par hare rang ke paani ki tarah dast jis me khoon aur luabiyat hoti hai:

a. Sign and symptoms of food poisoning

b. Sign and symptoms of Gastro enteritis

c. Sign and symptoms of Amoebiasis

d. Sign and symptoms of Cholera

162. Reham hewan ke pett me ek hewan hai kis ka Qaul hai:

a. Buqraat

b. Jalinoos

c. Aflatoon

d. Raazi

163. Zakkaria Rhazi advised it application in para umbilical region for Nutoo-e-Reham:

a. Rose water

b. Roghan-e-Gul

c. Aqaqia

d. All of the above

164. Reproductive organs me genital tuberculosis ki aam wajah hai:
a. Direct spread
b. Lymphatic spread
c. Both a & b
d. Haematogenous

165. In which parts of reproductive organs Peg cells are found:
a. Vagina
b. Vulva
c. Fallopian tubes
d. Ovary

166. Incubation period of Rubella is:
a. 3-4 days
b. 8-10 days
c. 14-21 days
d. 3-4 weeks

167. What is quantity of liquor in Polyhydramnios:
a. More than 1000ml
b. More than 500ml
c. More than 2000ml
d. More than 1500ml

168. Oestradiol ki peak ovulation hai:
a. Increase before 12-15 hours
b. Increase after 12-15 hours
c. Increase before 24-36 hours
d. Decrease after 24-3 6 hours

169. Hammam is advisable during:
a. Early pregnancy
b. Mid pregnancy
c. Late pregnancy

d. Few days before delivery

170. Best seasons for Fitaam is:
a. Summer
b. Winter
c. Autum
d. Both a & b

171. According to the Author of Alqanoon if a male baby is delivered puerperium lasts for:
a. Not more than 20 days
b. Not more than 25 days
c. Not more than 30 days
d. Not more than 35 days

172. Labour pain lasting for four days with difficulty in delivery is usually indicative of:
a. IUGR
b. APH
c. IUD
d. None of the above

173. Abnormal placenta ki wah kaun se halat hai jis me fetal blood loss hota hai:
a. Placenta praevia
b. Vasa paraveia
c. Placenta circumvallate
d. Placenta membranicaaea

174. Anaencephaly foetus aam taur par hote hai:
a. 70% females
b. 70% males
c. 30% females
d. 30 males

175. Braxton Hicks contractions in abdominal pregnancy:
a. Not felt
b. Felt
c. Disappear
d. None

176. Gestational hypertention hota hai
a. Without proteinuria
b. With proteinuria
c. Without convulsion
d. With convulsion

177. Patrogram ke zariye kis chheez ka record rakha jata hai:
a. Mareeza ka blood pressure
b. Mareeza ki nabz
c. Progress of labour
d. Foetal heart rate

178. Nose and mouth me white froath kis zehar me milte hai:
a. Dhatura
b. Opium
c. Castor
d. Croton

179. Incubation period of Mumps is:
a. 1-2 Weeks
b. 2-3 Weeks
c. 3-4 Weeks
d. 4-5 Weeks

180. Khandani mansooba bandi ke tahat mania hamal ke physical barrier tareeqo me darjai zail shamil hai:
a. Condom

b. Diaphram

c. Sponge

d. IUD

181.Daily requirement of calcium is:

a. 60 gram

b. 600 miligram

c. 60 miligram

d. 600gram

182. What is percentage of salt in oceans water?

a. 1.5

b. 2.5

c. 3.5

d. 4.5

183. Ahtabas ghair tabai darje zail sabab se nahi hota hai:

a. Quwwat zaeef ho jai

b. Majari tang wa masdood ho jai

c. Quwwate masika kamzoor ho jai

d. Quwwate hazima zaeef ho jai

184. Darje zail roghans me sab se ziyadah essential fatty acids kismet paya jata hai:

a. Safflower

b. Sun flower

c. Sesame

d. Mustard

185. Which of the following disease is not caused by folate deficiency?

a. Megaloblastic anaemia

b. Diarrhoea

c. Infertility

d. Peripheral neuritis

186. Kuon ki safai me paani ki miqdar maaloom karne ke liyer kaun sa formula correct hai?
a. 3.14xdxh/4)x1000
b, $3.14xd^2xh^2/4)x1000$
c. $3.14xd^2xh/4)x100$
d. $3.14xd^2xh/4)x1000$

187. Kis size ki gard (dust) Pneumoconiosis ke liye responsible hai?
a. 0.5-3micron
b. 0.5-3mm
c. 3-5 micron
d. 3-5 mm

188. Hammam ke teshre kamre ki kaifiat kiya honi chhaiye?
a. Motadil
b. Garam tar
c. Garam khusk
d. Sard khusk

189. The age of individual upto 25 years can be determined: from
a. Teeth
b. Ossification of bone
c. Height and weight
d. All of the above

190. The term death as commonly employed means:
a. Cellular death
b. Molecular death
c. Both a & b
d. Somatic death

191. Burking is a form of:
a. Asphyxia
b. Hanging
c. Strangulation
d. Drowning

192. Black eyes are cased due to:
a. Infra orbital hemorrhage
b. Supra orbital hemorrhage
c. Both a & b
d. None of the above

193. The most commonly employed chemical test to determine the presence of blood in the stain is:
a. Ortholidine test
b. Benzidine test
c. Both a & b
d. Locard test

194. Sui poison me shamil hai
a. Abrus precatorius
b. Dhatura
c. Opium
d. All of the above

195. Road poison is known as:
a. Dhatura
b. Castor
c. Croton
d. Nux vomica

196. Which of the following is the cause of cardiac arrest?
a. Nux vomica
b. Abrus precatotius
c. Digitalis

d. Opium

197. In which poisoning green color vomiting occurs?
a. Iodine
b. Cannabis
c. Copper sulphate
d. Carbon tetra chloride

198. Tetanus is caused by:
a. Clostridium welchi
b. Staphylococcus albus
c. E. coli
d. Clostridium tetani

199.The cause of smell may be due to:
a. Ammonia
b. Indole
c. Skatole
d. All of the above

200. Duodenal ulcer is more common in:
a. Posterior part of duodenum
b. First part of duodenum
c. Second part of duodenum
d. Anterior part of duodenum

MD AMU ENTRANCE EXAMNATION ANSWER KEY 2013-14

1. B	2. B	3. C	4. A	5. C
6. B	7. C	8. C	9. C	10. C
11. D	12. C	13. B	14. D	15. B
16. A	17. A	18. D	19. D	20. A
21. B	22. C	23. A	24. A	25. B
26. D	27. B	28. A	29. B	30. A
31. C	32. B	33. A	34. C	35. C
36. B	37. D	38. C	39. C	40. A
41. D	42. A	43. B	44. D	45. A
46. A	47. B	48. A	49. A	50. B
51. A	52. A	53. A	54. A	55. B
56. C	57. D	58. A	59. B	60. C
61. B	62. C	63. B	64. B	65. B
66. C	67. A	68. B	69. A	70. A
71. C	72. A	73. A	74. B	75. C
76. D	77. C	78. D	79. C	80. C
81. C	82. D	83. A	84. A	85. B
86. B	87. A	88. D	89. A	90. D
91. A	92. B	93. C	94. C	95. D
96. B	97. D	98. A	99. C	100. B
101. A	102. A	103. B	104. A	105. D
106. C	107. D	108. B	109. D	110. C
111. C	112. C	113. A	114. C	115. B
116. C	117. A	118. B	119. A	120. C
121. B	122. A	123. B	124. C	125. A
126. D	127. D	128. B	129. C	130. C
131. A	132. B	133. D	134. C	135. B
136. C	137. B	138. C	139. D	140. B
141. C	142. D	143. D	144. B	145. D
146. A	147. D	148. A	149. D	150. A
151. C	152. A	153. A	154. D	155. C
156. B	157. A	158. B	159. C	160. C
161.B	162.C	163.C	164.D	165. C

166.C 167.C 168.C 169.D 170. C
171.C 172.C 173.B 174.A 175. A
176.A 177.C 178.B 179.B 180. D
181.B 182.C 183.C 184.A 185. D
186.D 187.A 188.C 189.D 190. D
191.A 192.B 193.B 194.D 195. A
196.C 197.A 198.D 199.D 200. B

1. Glomerular Hydrostatic pressure is depends on which of the following factor:
a. On arterial pressure
b. On afferent arteriolar resistance
c. On efferent arteriolar resistance
d. All of the above

2. Which clinical features are present in Parkinson's disease?
a. Rigidity
b. Involuntary tremor
c. Difficulty in initiating the movement of body
d. All of the above

3. Which of the following statement is correct?
a. Sympathetic stimulation se basal metabolism me izafa ho jata hai
b. Sympathetic stimulation se basal metabolism me kami ho jata hai
c. Sympathetic stimulation se basal metabolism par koi faraq nahi parta hai
d. Parasympathetic stimulation se basal metabolism me izafa ho jata hai

4. The new growth of B.V me izafa kis factors ki waja se hota hai:
a. Vascular endothelial growth factor
b. Fibroblast growth factor
c. Angiogenin
d. All of the above

5. Which statement is correct about Myasthenia Gravis?
a. Caused by Myasthenia virus
b. It is an infectious disease
c. It is an autoimmune disease
d. All of the above

6. In which of the following condition edema is caused:
a. Increased capillary pressure
b. Decreased plasma protein
c. Increased capillary permeability
d. All of the above

7. What is done in Ataxia?
a. Uncoordinated movement
b. Fast coordinated movement
c. Slow coordinated movement
d. No movement

8. Which coagulating factors is not synthesized during deficiency of Vit. K?
a. Prothrombin
b. Factor VII
c. Factor IX
d. None of the above

9. Best method of sterilization is:
a. Hot air oven
b. Autoclave
c. Steam
d. Inspissator

10. Maximum body water is present:
a. Extracellular
b. Intracellular
c. Intravascular

d. Equal a and b

11. Fate of thrombosis is:
a. Resolution
b. Organization
c. Propagation & Thromboembolism
d. All of the above

12. Passive Hyperemia is the result of:
a. Dilation of capillaries
b. Dilation of arterioles
c. Impaired venous drainage
d. Lymphatic

13. Sua-e-Mizaj Mustavi me:
a. Dard ka ehsaas dafattan hota hai
b. Dard ka ehsaaskabhi hota hai Dard ka ehsaas dafattan hita hai
c. Dard ka ehsaas kabhi nahi hota hai
d. Dard ka ehsaas mustaqil hota hai

14. Keloid is:
a. Scar due to burn
b. Recurrent fibroblastic tumor
c. Excessive collagen accumulation
d. None of the above

15. Necrosis in brain is commonly:
a. Coagulative
b. Caseous
c. Liquefactive
d. Enzymatic

16. Between CO and O2 hemoglobin has:
a. Greater affinity for CO
b. Greater affinity for O2

c. Equal affinity for both
d. None is correct

17. Cloudy Swelling commonly found in:
a. Liver
b. Kidney
c. Heart
d. All of the above

18. Line of Zahn occur in
a. Postmortem clot
b. Infarct
c. Embolus
d. Coraline Thrombus

19. Foreign body giant cells have:
a. Upto 100 nuclei
b. Arranged in the periphery
c. Vacuolated cytoplasm
d. Derived from cardiac histocyles

20. Sighr-ul-Saddi ka sabab hai:
a. Saddi ki quwwat-e-Jazba ka zaeef hona
b. Saddi ko jane wali shiryaan me sudda
c. Kasrate thalul wa istifragh se badan me khushki wa fasade khoon ka hona
d. All of the above

21. Sheer Gao Sheerzan ke muqable me:
a. Lateef aur zoodhazam hota hai
b. Ghaleez aur der hazam hota hai
c. Lateff lekin der hazam hota hai
d. Ghaleez lekin zoodhazam

22. Cervix ke smear ko kis ke zariye liya jata hai
a. Cotton swab

b. Spatula
c. Pipette
d. Glass slide

23. In which condition hormonal replacement therapy prohibited?
a. Vasomotor symptoms
b. Urogenital atrophy
c. Estrogen dependent neoplasm
d. Colorectal carcinoma

24. What is the classical symptom's of Fibroid?
a. Menorrhagia
b. Metrorhagia
c. Polymenorrhoea
d. DUB

25. In normal Women at what percentages of incidence of retroversion:
a. 5-10%
b. 15-20%
c. 30-35%
d. 5%

26. In vestibule how much opening is present:
a. 1
b. 2
c. 3
d. 4

27. Gardan reham agar baghair salabat ke band hai to:
a. This sign of pregnancy
b. This sign of abortion
c. This sign of cancer
d. This sign of inflammation

28. In leucorrhoea which quwwat is week?
a. Quwwate namia
b. Quwwate ghazia
c. Quwwate masika
d. Both a & b

29. All are the cause of Asymmetrical IUGR except:
a. Intrauterine infection
b. Cigarettes smoking
c. Inborn error of metabolism
d. Anemia

30. After delivery how much follicles are present in single ovary:
a.1-2 Million
b. 2-3 Million
c. 3-4 Million
d. 4-5 Million

31. Gonads ki tafreeque ki in ko ovary banna hai ya testes mouqamal ho jati hai:
a. In5- 9th gestational weeks
b. In 6-9th gestational weeks
c. In6- 11th gestational weeks
d. In 8-10th gestational weeks

32. All are the probable sign of the pregnancy except:
a. Softening of the cervix
b. Braxton Hicks contraction
c. Abdominal enlargement
d. Quickening

33. Shaqaqur Reham ki waja hai:
a. Removal of fetus suddenly
b. Removal of placent suddenly
c. M.C comes suddenly

d. All of the above

34. Conception is not done if:
a. If excess baroodat and kasafat in reham
b. If excess baroodat
c. If excess hararat
d. All of the above

35. The following statements regarding the portal vein are correct except the:
a. It is formed by the superior mesenteric and inferior mesenteric veins
b. It opens into the porta hepatic
c. The superiorpancreatico duodenal veins open directly in to it
d. It has right and left hepatic branches

36. The following structures pass through greater sciatic foramen except:
a. Superior gluteal artery
b. Tendon of obturator internus
c. Sciatic nerve
d. Pudendal nerve

37. About the neuron it is true except that:
a. It is the functional and Structural unit of the body
b. It has axon which conduct impulses towards the cell body
c. It has dendrites which contain nissl bodies
d. It is a cell body with a large nucleus

38. The following nerves are directly related to the humerus except the:
a. Ulnar nerve
b. Median nerve

c. Axillary nerve
d. Radial nerve

39. Regarding the descending thoracic aorta it is true except that:
a. It is continuation of arch of aorta
b. It passes through aortic opening of diaphragm at the level of 8th thoracic vertebra
c. The posterior intercostals arteries arise from it
d. It lies throughout in the posterior mediastinum

40. The following structures lie in front of the right kidney except the:
a. Liver
b. Pancreas
c. Duodenum
d. Right suprarenal gland

41. The facial nerve emerges from the skull through:
a. Foramen ovale
b. Foramen spinosum
c. Stylomastoid foramen
d. Zygomaticofacial foramen

42. The facial nerve supplies the following muscles except
a. All muscles of the facial expression
b. All muscles of mastication
c. Stapedius
d. Stylohyoid

43. GOBI Compaign is related with:
a. WHO
b. UNDP
c. UNICEF

d. USAID

44. Milk borne disease is:
a. Tuberculosis
b. Brucellosis
c. Salmonellosis
d. All of the above

45. Cardiac beriberi is related with which types of beriberi:
a. Dry
b. Wet
c. Infantile
d. Senile

46. Three Ds Diarrhoea, dermatitis and dementia is related with:
a. Riboflavin
b. Thiamine
c. Niacin
d. Pyridoxine

47. Muarique Advia ke ubalte hoae joshandah ki bhaap se paseena lane ko kiya kahte hain?
a. Bakhoor
b. Inkabab
c. Takmeed
d. Poltis

48. Neend poori na hone ke sabab Aayai ki kaun se qism lahique hogi?
a. Aayai Qazfi
b. Aayai Farohi
c. Aayai Tamaddudi
d. Aayai Warmi

49. Hammam ke aakhri kamre ki hawa kaisi honi chhahiye?
a. Garam khushk
b. Garam tar
c. Sard khushk
d. Sard tar

50. Hawai muheet -e-Rooh ke tabai mizaj ke muqable:
a. Ziyadah barid hoti hai
b. Kam barid hoti hai
c. Ziyadah haar hoti hai
d. Kam haar hoti hai

51. Al Hawia wal miah wal Joodyah (air, water and places) naam ki kitab kis ne likhi?
a. Ibn-e-Sina
b. Hoppocrate
c. Asqaliboos
d. Jalinoos

52. In disinfection which rays are used:
a. Gamma rays
b. Alpha rays
c. X- rays
d. None of the above

53. Diarrhea is most common at what age groups?
a. 10-15 years
b. 3-5 years
c. 6 month to 2 years
d. After 6 month of birth

54. Kis umr me Hajamat se parhaiz bataya gaya hai?
a. Less than 10 years
b. More than 60 years
c Less than 10 years and more than 60 years
d. None of the above

55. How much energy is obtained from one gram of carbohydrate?
a. 4kcal
b. 4cal
c. 40cal
d. 40kcl

56. Apoplexy ki sorat me imala ki kaun se qism ka intikhab kare gai?
a. Imala qareeb
b. Imala baieed
c. Imala qareeb and baieed
d. None of the above

57. For prevention of pellagra which is used?
a. Use of fruits
b. Use of vegetables
c. Different types of oils
d. Use of milk and meats

58. Reactionary hemorrhage occurs:
a. At the time of surgery
b. Due to reaction of drugs
c. After 10-12 days of surgery
d. After 8-10 hours of surgery

59. Dukes staging is done to classified:
a. Fistula in ano
b. Different types of burns
c. Spread of carcinoma of rectum
d. Stages of Carcinoma head of pancreas

60. Which of the following is the most effective intravesical therapy for superficial bladder cancer?
a. Mitonmycin

b. Adriamycin
c. Thiotepa
d. BCG

61. Bradycardia is common after injection of:
a. Midazolam
b. Succinyl Choline
c. Dopamine
d. Isoprenaline

62. Deep inguinal ring is situated in:
a. Internal oblique muscle
b. Transverse abdominis
c. Internal spermatic fascia
d. Transversalis fascia

63. Which of the following bone tumors typically affects the epiphysis of long bone?
a. Osteosarcoma
b. Ewing's sarcoma
c. Chodroblastoma
d. Chondromyxoid

64. All of the following diseases cause massive spleenomegaly except?
a. Malaria
b. Kalazar
c. Lymphoblastic leukemia
d. Idiopathic myelofibrosis

65. The first person to advocate the use of compression bandage to treat leg ulcer was:
a. Ibn-e-Sina
b. Hippocrates
c. C.C. Michel
d. Abul Qasim Zohrawi

66. The ratio of O2 and N2O given during general anesthesia is usually:
a. 33:67
b. 67:33
c. 60:40
d. 10:90

67. The commonest site of cancer of colon is:
a. Rectum
b. Caecum
c. Ascending colon
d. Descending colon

68. The complication of Ulcerative colitis:
a. Acute toxic dilation
b. Perforation
c. Hemorrhage
d. All of the above

69. Temporary colostomy kis jagah banai ja sakti hai:
a. Left upper quadrant
b. Right upper quadrant
c. Right iliac fossa
d. Left iliac fossa

70. Least common position of appendix is:
a. Retroileal
b. Retrocoecal
c. Postileal
d. Pelvic

71. The cause of Hashimotos thyroiditis:
a. Bacterial infection
b. Viral infection
c. Autoimmune disease
d. Fungal infection

72. Breast conservation surgery me kam se kam kitne axillary lyphnode ko sample karna chhaiye?
a. 2
b. 3
c. 4
d. 5

73. In which part of stomach the cancer is commonest?
a. Pyloric
b. Cardiac
c. Greater curvature
d. None of the above

74. Oshdners clasping test is done for:
a. Appendicitis
b. Cholecystitis
c. Median nerve testing
d. Ulnar nerve testing

75. Which of the following is not an intravenous anaesthetic agent?
a. Isoflurane
b. Propofol
c. Etomidate
d. Methohexitone

76. Heel khurad is:
a. Fruit
b. Flower
c. Buds
d. Zaydah ba sabab kiram

77. Mufareh-e-Shaikhur Rais ka main ingredient hai:
a. Murvareed
b. Dronaj aqrabi
c. Gaozabah

d. Abresham

78. Which of the following drug is not updhat?
a. Darchikna
b. Raskapoor
c. Gandhak
d. Abrak

79. Kaknaj hindi ka mutradif hai:
a. Kaknaj
b. Asgand
c. Makko
d. None of the above

80. Safoof-e-Imlah ka main ingredient is:
a. Khar bhang
b. Khar Moli
c. Khar poodina
d.Khar chirchitta

81. Anooshdaroo ka doosra nam hai:
a. Majoon jalinoos
b. Majoon kindi
c. Majoon zabeeb
d. Majoon shikam seer

82. Kaun se dawa muqawwi bah ashar nahi rakhti hai?
a. Khusta jamun
b. Saalab mishri
c. Shaqaqil mishri
d. Satawar

83. Rakhu bafrat kis ki ki qism hai?
a. Mizaj saani mustahkam ki
b. Mizaj saani ghair mustahkam ki
c. Rakhu mutlaq ki
d. Rakhu zidan

84. Lodh pathani ka kaun sa juz dawa ke taur par use hota hai?
a. Root
b. Flower
c. Post
d. Shagofa

85. Qayasi aetibar se hareef dawa ka mizaj hota hai:
a. Matowast garam aur zyadah khusk
b. Zyadah garam aur Matowast khusk
c. Zyadah garam aur kam khusk
d. Motadil aur zyadah khusk

86. Kanocha ka kaun sa juz dawa ke taur par use hota hai?
a. Tukhm
b. Flower
c. Root
d. All of the above

87. Kushta shangaraf miyaari samjha jata hai:
a. Agar use aag par dale to dhua na de
b. Agar ise arqe limou me kharal kare to is ka rang na tabdeel ho
c. Both of the above
d. None of the above

88. Which drug having garam khusk temperament?
a. Sadaf marvareed
b. Sadaf Halzoon
c. Sadaf Kharmohra
d. All of the above

89. Majoon Mughaliz ka main ingredient hai:
a. Saalab mishri

b. Fandaq

c. Maghz Badam

d. Panba dana

90. Kaun sa tareeka ziyadah hararat paida karta hai?
a. Bhandh patth
b. Bajar path
c. Barah path
d. Ganj path

91. Samagh arabi, kateera and Jao sheer group ki dawa hai:
a. Organized
b. Unorganized
c. Plants and animals
d. None of the above

92. Papaver somniferum se hasil shudah chemical substance hai:
a. Morphine
b. Codeine
c. Thebane
d. All of the above

93. Sate gillo kis plants se hasil hota hai?
a. Tinospora cardifolia
b. Sida cardifolia
c. Cuscuta reflexa
d. Cuscuta chinensis

94. Crocus sativus Linn is the botanical name of:
a. Seer
b. Kurkum
c. Sumaq
d. Sheetraj hindi

95. Baid anjeer me paya jane wala zahareela maddah kaun hai?
a. Atropine
b. Cycasine
c. Aconitine
d. Ricin

96. Husne yusuf ka kaun sa hissa mustamil hai:
a. Tukhm
b. Barg
c. Flower
d. Gond

97. Tarpeen ka oil kis palnt se hasil kiya jata hai:
a. Cedar deodara
b. Juniper communis
c. Ephedra sinica
d. Pinus polustris

98. Qatile deedan aama dawa ki nishandahi kare?
a. Tukhm dhakh
b. Damul akhwain
c. Habb-ul-Qatan
d. Kiram arosak

99. Kis Zaiqah ki Advia tafteh arooq baas nahi hoti hain?
a. Murr
b. Afis
c. Maleh
d. Hareef

100. Bacchnag ka musleh kaun si dawa hai us ka naam nabati naam kiya hai?
a. Delphinium denudatum
b. Derris elliptica

c. Aconitum hetrophllum

d. Aconitum napellus

101. In which of the following drug all parts are used as a medicinal?

a. Ushr

b. Chandan booti

c. Nissoot

d. Pakhan baid

102. What is shelf life of gum?

a. I year

b. 2 years

c. 3 years

d. 4years

103. Ajmaleen alkaloid kis dawa se alaihidah kiya jata hai?

a. Yabrojulsanam

b. Chandan booti

c. Asganh

d. Ajwain khurasani

104. What is the botanical name of Asganh nagori?

a. Rauwolfia serpentine

b. Solanum tuberosum

c. Solanum niger

d. Withania somnifera

105. Aatees ka kaun sa hissa mustamil hai?

a. Whole plant

b. Root

c. Fruits

d. Tukhm

106. Alqanoon fit Tib me Qarabadeen par mushtamil jild kaun si hai?
a. Volume I
b. Volume III
c. Volume IV
d. Volume

107.Which is the most toxic effect of NSAIDs (e.g Aspirin)?
a. Kidney damage
b. Teratogenic effects
c. Gastric toxicity
d. Aplastic anemia

108. Which of the following drugs is most effective in suppressing acid secretion in peptic ulcer?
a. Proton pump inhibitors
b. H2- Antagonist
c. Sucralfate
d. Antacids

109. Given by slow injection:
a. Diazoxide
b. Xylocaine
c. Aminophylline
d. Hydrocortisone

110. A patient receiving following drugs developed facial muscle dystonia. Which drug is the:
a. Dextropropoxyphene
b. Antacids
c. Metachlopramide
d. Omeprazole

111. Prevent reinfarction after myocardial infarction:
a. Diuretics

b. Morphine

c. Diazepam

d. Beeta blockers

112. Which is the most likely adverse effect of Streptomycin?

a. Nephrotoxicity

b. Hepatotixicity

c. Ophthalmic toxicity

d. Peripheral neuropathy

113. Which of the following is commonly used dose of aspirin for prevention of thrombosis?

a. 500mg

b. 150mg

c. 300mg

d. 75mg

114. Which of the common adverse effect of anti muscarinic agent like Atopine, Ipratropium etc?

a. Renal failure

b. Vomiting

c. Dry mouth

d. Abdominal pain

115. A person sensitive to penicillin may also be sensitive to which of the following?

a. Cephalosporin

b. Tetracycline

c. Aminoglycosides

d. Quinolones

116. Which of the following is the dangerous toxic effect of Parcetamol overdose?

a. Liver failure

b. Kidney failure

c. Stroke

d. MI

117. Artemether may produce which of the following adverse effects?

a. Nausea and vomiting

b. Neurotoxicity

c. Blindness

d. Renal failure

118. Spontaneous pneumothorax is seen in:

a. Smokers

b. Old age

c. During exercise

d. Children

119. Hasham kahte hai:

a. Quwwate shamia ka madoom hona

b. Quwwate shamia ka bigarh

c. Fasaad khasham

d. All of above

120. Safoofe muqliyaha ka main ingredient hai:

a. Sauneez

b. Zafran

c. Tukhm Haloon

d. None of the above

121. Ibn-e-Sina kis muqam ke bashindo ko motadil mizaj kahte hai?

a. Khate istawa

b. Khate sartan

c. Khate jiddi

d. Qutube junoobi

122. Khoon ka mizaj kis unsure ke mizaj ke mutradif hai:

a. Hawa

b. Water

c. Naar

d. None of the above

123. Aazai Murakkaba ka degar nam kiya hai:

a. Aazai raisa

b. Aazai Aalia

c. Aazai shumara

d. Aazai tabaiyah

124. Maddah mani ko uzu ki shakal ikhtiyar karwane me kaun se quwwqt maun hai?

a. Quwwate ghazia

b. Quwwate namia

c. Quwwate molidah

d. Quwwate masauwira

125. Ahmar nasah aur haad kaun se khilt hai:

a. Safara tabai

b. Safara ghair tabai

c. Mirrah safara

d. Safara muhayah

126. Which of the following kaifiyat is known as kaifiyate faila?

a. Hararat wa ratoobat

b. Hararat wa yabusat

c. Ratoobat wa yabusat

d. Hararat wa yabusat

127. Rabat ka shumaar kis me hota hai?

a. Aazai harra

b. Aazai barida

c. Aazai yabisa

d. Aazai ratba

128. Amale taghzia me kaun si quwwat pahle amal karti hai:

a. Quwwat-e-masika

b. Quwwat-e-hazma

c. Quwwat-e-dafia

d. Quwwat-e-jaziba

129. Kis group ke mutabique anasir ki tadad four hai?

a. Ashabe khaleet

b. Falasfa mashain

c. Ahle akseer

d. None of the above

130. Tabai maut mizaj awwal ke mutabique waqai hoti hai:

a. Raban Tabri

b. Zakaria Razi

c. Ibne Sina

d. Hakeem Ajmal Khan

131. Kitabul kuliyat ke Author ka name hai:

a. Ibn-e-Rushd

b. Ibn-e-Nafis

c. Raseed mohammad kamaluddin Husain hamdani

d. Abusahal masihi

132. Tashkhees mizaj ke liye ajnas-e-ushrah ka zikr kis ne kiya hai?

a. Zakaria Razi

b. Ali Ibne Abbas majoosi

c. Ibne Sina

d. Abu Sahal masihi

133. Hisse Mushtarak ke zariya kin quwwato ka istarak hota hai?

a. Quwwate hissia wa quwwate muharika

b. Hawase khamsa zahira

c. Hawase khamsa batina

d. All of the above

134. Quwwate Shokia ka fail kiya hai?

a. Harkat

b. Hiss

c. Samaat

d. Inhamak

135. Hazoom-e-arba ke tahat hazme kabdi kaun sa hazam hai?

a. First

b. second

c. Thrird

d. Fourth

36. Aazai Raisa me kaun sa uzu shamil hai?

a. Qalb

b. Brain

c. Kidney

d. Kabid

137. Maze ke lihaz se balgham gair tabai ki kitni qisme hain?

a. 4

b. 2

c. 3

d. 5

138. Baqai naaui kelihaz se Aazai Raisa ki tadaa kitni hai?

a. 1

b. 2

c. 3

d. 5

139. Khilti ratoobat ke fana hone ko ka khas zariya kiya hai?

a. Taareeque

b. Badal ma tahalul

c. Hararat-e-Ghareeba

d. Idrare boul

140. Kaun se khilt khoon ko lateef banati hai aur tang raston me nafooz karati hai?

a. Khoon

b. Safra

c. Balgham

d. Sauda

141. Khoon ka mizaj kis fasal ke mizaj se mushabah hota hai?

a. Fasal-e-Khareef

b. Fasal-e-Saif

c. Fasal-e-Shita

d. Fasal-e-Rabih

142. Marz Ilattul zaib ka mutradif hai:

a. Mania

b. Melancholia

c. Qutrub

d. Daul qalb

143. Balihaz baqai naau quwwa zarooriya kitne hai?

a. 2

b. 3

c. 4

d. 5

144. Which of the following book is not written by Ibne Sina?
a. Kitabul tabiyatul Insan
b. Kitabul shifa
c. Kitabul najat
d. Cannon of medicine

145. Balgham ki khas sifat kiya hai:
a. Badan ko garam rakhna
b. Khoon ko aaza me nafooz karana
c. Safra ke qawam ko motadil rakhna
d. Qilat-e-dam ki soorat me khoon ka badal ban jana

146. Fataq kiya hai?
a. Andarooni uzu ka tabai soorakh se bahar aana
b. Andarooni uzu ka gair tabai soorakh se bahar aana
c. Andarooni uzu ka kisi shigaf se bahar aana
d. All of the above

147. Kis Qoolinj me stomach ko dabane par dard nahi hota hai?
a. Qoolin warmi
b. Qoolin imtali
c. Qoolin rehi
d. Qoolin iltavai

148. Qitmaa kahte hai:
a. Sirf gahri siyahi ko
b. Surkhi ke saath siyahi ko
c. Surkhi ke saath nele pan ko
d. All of the above

149. Istalahan lafz Zaghott ka mutradif hai:
a. Marz Ishque
b. Marz kaboos

c. marz kashratulnauum

d. None of the above

150. Gurde me pathri paida hone ke liye do chhezai zaroori hain ghaliz maddah aur ghaliz maddah ka rukna kis ka qaul hai?

a. Buqraat

b, Jalinoos

c. Zakaria Razi

d. Shaikh bo ali sina

151. Dard ba sabab hisathul-kuliya ko aaram milta hai:

a. Fasad keefa

b. Fasad char rag

c. Fasad basleeq

d. None of the above

152. Marz Sibara ka sabab hai:

a. Safrawi dam muharique

b. Safrawi sauda muharique

c. Balghami sauda muharique

d. Dam muharique

153. Arad halia aur sheerazia tibbi nuqte nazar se kis ki aqsaam hain?

a. Kasarul azam ki

b. Rasooliyo ki

c. Ghudad aqad ki

d. Auram aur basoor ki

154. Tarasiyoos dar asal saaleel ki vah qism hai:

a. Jin ki gahrai me peep bhari hoti hai

b. Jin ke sire mekhoon ke manind hote hai

c. Jin ke moh andar ke janib gaust me piyost hote hai

d. Jo ressadar hote hai

155. Jab sar ki jild me bareek bareek soorakh ho jate hain aur unke moh par zarad aab bhara hota hoa maloom hota hai to un ko tibbi istalah me kiya kaha jata hai:
a. Sufa Humarah
b. Sufa taini
c. Sufa shadiya
d. None of the above

156. Nafas muzaaif paya jata hai:
a. Buhar me
b. Zatur riya
c. Dabba itifal
d. All of the above

157. Rasha paida hota hai:
a. Aazai mufarda me
b. Aazai murakkab me
c. Both a and b
d. None of the above

158. Alamat-e-Munzara ka taaluque kis qism ki suda se hai?
a. Suda shaqeeqa
b. Suda Baiza khoza
c. Suda Shirki madi
d. Suda Khimari

159. Saraa ki qism me shamil nahi hai:
a. Saraa madi
b. Saraa deedani
c. Saraa shirki
d. Saraa khumari

160. Qutrub ek marz hai jis me mareez:
a. Jugno ke manind be tarteeb aur tez harkate karta hai

b, Khamoosh rahta hai

c. Chekhta hai

d. Kutto ke manind harkat karta hai

161. Jigar ke maqar hissa me sudde par jatte hain:

a. Lesdar gizaon ke bakashrat istamal se

b. Mirch wa masalh ke kasarat istemal se

c. Khan eke baad ziyadah miqdar me paani peene se

d. Jima ki kasrat se

162. Siyah yarqan paida hota hai:

a. Jigar wa Tihal ke mauf hone kise

b. Jigar me suddah lahiq hone se

c. Tihal me suddah lahiq hone se

d. Tihal me waram hone se

163. Sab se ziyadah hummiyat ki istidad hoti hai:

a. Harr ratab mizaj walon me

b. Harr yabis mizaj walon me

c. Barid ratab mizaj walon me

d. Barid yabis mizaj walon me

164. Zoosantaria safarawi me:

a. Aanto me dard hota hai

b. Stomach o me dard hota hai

c. Jigar me dard hota hai

d. Miqad me dard hota hai

165. Humme mukhtalta paya jata hai:

a. Warme kuliya haad

b. Sarsam haar me

c. Warme kabid haar

d. Warme masana

166. Silk e mareez ke liye umdah dawa hai:

a. Sartan nuhri

b. Majoon Aqrab

c. Majoon Nankhuah

d. Majoon Piyaz

167. Sarsam-e-Harr Me zubaan hoti hai:

a. Mukaddir

b. Saaf

c. Zardi mail

d. Surkh

168. Damwi Bukhar ko kahte hain:

a. Humm-e- Mutbaka

b. Humm-e- Ghib

c. Humm-e- Mawaziba

d. Humm-e- Dairah

169. Most common symptoms of carcinoma of lung is:

a. Chest pain

b. Dyspnoea

c. Weight loss

d. Cough

170. Mani ki hiddat me mufeed hai:

a. Khurfa

b. Zeerah siyah

c. Shoneez

d. Tukhm hulbah

171. Hissate gurdah banne ka faili sabab hai:

a. Hararat

b. Ghaliz maddah

c. Hazal-e-Kuliya

d. Infection of urethra

172. Synonyms of syphilis is:

a. Saaoor

b. Zarma

c. Batam

d. Both a & b

173. Umme dimagh kise kahte hai:
a. Umme ghaliz

b. Umme raqeeq

c. Ghisai ankabooti

d. All of the above

174. Clubbing of finger is not seen:
a. Bronchiectesis

b. Empyema

c. Pneumonia

d. Emphysema

175. What is not happened in the hypokalemia?
a. Abdominal distention

b. Vomiting

c. Muscles weakness

d. Increased peristalsis

176. Comedones are found in?
a. Acne vulgaris

b. Psoriasis

c. Lichen planus

d. None of the above

177. Quwwat-e-Mudafiat me barah-e-rast amal dakhil hai:
a. Thymus gland

b. Thyroid gland

c. Pancreas

d. None of the above

178. Cause of Urticaria:
a. Skin allergy

b. Gut allergy

c. Infection

d. Vitamins deficiency

179. Which leprosy is most infectious?

a. Indeterminate H.D

b. Paucibacillary H.D

c. Multibacilarry H.D

d. Neuritic H.D

180. Cause of Zollinger Ellision Syndrome:

a. Gastrinoma

b. Pseudopancreatic cyst

c. Hepatoma

d. None of the above

181. Deficiency of Iron level in except?

a. Anemia due to chronic infection

b. Sideroblastic anemia

c. Anemia due to peptic ulcer

d. Iron deficiency of anemia

182. The tumor maker of Hepatocellular carcinoma:

a. A.F.P

b. H.C.G

c. C.E.A

d. C.A-125

183. Stooped Gait is found in:

a. Hemiplegia

b. Paraplegia

c. Parkinsonism

d. Brain tumor

184. Piebaldism is found in which disease?

a. Fungal infection of skin

b. Eczema of skin

c. Albinism

d. None of the above.

185. What is lower motor neuron?
a. Cells of cerebral cortex

b. Anterior horn of spinal cord

c. Posterior horn of spinal cord

d. Caudate nucleus

186. Blood gas analysis is done in which blood?
a. Arterial blood

b. Venous blood

c. Capillary blood

d. All of them

187. What is seen in Thoracoscopy?
a. Bronchial tree

b. Pleural cavity

c. Thoracic cavity

d. Alveoli of lungs

188. Cardiac output is depend on:
a. Peripheral resistance

b. Diameter of aorta

c. Stroke volume

d. Atrial contraction

189. What is characteristic presenting feature of osteoarthritis?
a. Pain

b. Swelling of joints

c. Redness of joints

d. Deformity

190. Innocent murmur is characteristic of:
a. Aortic regurgitation

b. Thyrotoxicosis

c. Mitral regurgitation
d. VSD

191. Pain that is produced by light touch or pressure is called:
a. Allodynia
b. Nocception
c. Hyperalgesia
d. Hypoaesthesia

192. Swan neck deformity is found in:
a. Rheumatic arthritis
b. Rheumatoid arthritis
c. Septic arthritis
d. None of the above

193. Grey Turners syndrome is found in which disease?
a. Myocarditis
b. Pancreatitis
c. Appendicitis
d. Cholecystitis

194. Amphoric bronchial breathing is seen in:
a. Pericardial effusion
b. Pleural effusion
c. Pneumothorax
d. Pneumonia

195. The cause of Monilial stomatitis:
a. Malnutrition
b. Candida albicans
c. Antamaeba gingivalis
d. All of the above

196. Varicella Zoster cuases:
a. Herpes zoster

b. Chicken pox
c. German measles
d. Both a & b

197. The importance of blood culture is more in:
a. Enteric fever
b. Infective endocarditis
c. Dengue fever
d. Both a & b

198. The hormones which is responsible for contraction of pregnant uterus:
a. Oxytocin
b. HCG
c. Both a & b
d. None of the above

199. In which mass discharge is occur?
a. Sympathetic system
b. Parasympathetic system
c. Both a & b
d. None of the above

200. Those drugs which acts on adrenergic effectors organ is known as:
a. Sympathomimetic
b. Parasympathomimetic
c. Anticholintesterase
d. Beta blockers

MD AMU ENTRANCE EXAMNATION
ANSWERS KEY 2012-13

1. D   2. D   3. A   4. D   5. C
6. D   7. A   8. D   9. B   10. B
11. D   12. C   13. C 14. C   15. C
16. A   17. D   18. D   19. A   20. D
21. B   22. B   23. C   24. A   25. B
26. D   27. A   28. B   29. D   30. A
31. B   32. D   33. D   34. D   35. A
36. B   37. B   38. B   39. B   40. B
41. C   42. B   43. C   44. D   45. A
46. C   47. B   48. C   49. A   50. A
51. B   52. A   53. C   54. C   55. A
56. C   57. D   58. D   59. C   60. D
61. B   62. D   63. C   64. C   65. B
66. A   67. A   68. D   69. B   70. A
71. C   72. C   73. A   74. C   75. A
76. A   77. B   78. D   79. B   80. B
81. B   82. A   83. B   84. C   85. B
86. A   87. C   88. C   89. C   90. B
91. B   92. D   93. A   94. B   95. D
96. A   97. D   98. A   99. B   100. A
101. A 102. C 103. B 104. D 105. B
106. D 107. C 108. A 109. C 110. C
111. D 112. A 113. D 114. C 115. A
116. A 117. A 118. A 119. A 120. C
121. A 122. A 123. B 124. B 125. A
126. D 127. B 128. D 129. B 130. C
131. A 132. C 133. B 134. A 135. B
136. C 137. A 138. D 139. C 140. B
141. A 142. C 143. C 144. A 145. D
146. D 147. C 148. B 149. B 150. D
151. C 152. B 153. B 154. D 155. C
156. B 157. B 158. A 159. C 160. A
161. A 162. A 163. A 164. A 165. A

166.A 167.A 168.A 169.D 170.A
171.A 172.D 173.B 174.C 175.D
176.A 177.A 178.B 179.C 180.A
181.B 182.A 183.C 184.C 185.B
186.A 187.B 188.C 189.A 190.B
191.A 192.B 193.B 194.C 195.B
196.D 197.D 198.A 199.A 200.A

MD AMU ENTRANCE EXAMNATION 2010-11

1. Iltihab-e-Ghisai ki soorat me qalb ki aawaaz:
a. Tez sunai deti hai
b. Normal se kam sunai deti hai
c. Qatai taur par sunai nahi deti hai
d. Aawaaz par koi faraq nahi parta hai

2. Corpulmonale ki ibtida hoti hai:
a. Qalb se hoti hai
b. Vareed se hoti hai
c. Artery se hoti hai
d. Aorta se hoti hai

3. Rh-incompatibility soote janeen ka rare cause hota hai hasbe zail muddat me:
a. 28 weeks
b. 24 weeks
c. 16 weeks
d. 12 weeks

4. Sukoone badni har halat me darje zail kaifiat paida karti hai:
a. Mubarid
b. Muratib
c. Mubarid and Muratib
d. None of the above

5. Which nerve is related to the surgical neck of humerus?
a. Axillary nerve
b. Radial nerve
c. Ulnar nerve
d. Median nerve

6. Laqwa ka ilaj:
a. Wajaul asaab ke usool par kiya jata hai
b. Falij ke usool par kiya jata hai
c. Sara ke usool par kiya jata hai
d. Sarsam ke usool par kiya jata hai

7. Marz kaboos:
a. Ek khilti marz hai
b. Ek asabi marz hai
c. Ek istihali marz hai
d. Ek mutaddi marz hai

8. Marz Faranitus:
a. Khilte dam ke fasad se hota hai
b. Khilte safra ke fasad se hota hai
c. Khilte balgham ke fasad se hota hai
d. Khilte sauda ke fasad se hota hai

9. Kernings sign is found in which disease?
a. Sarsam balghami
b. Marz Sara
c. Ikhtanaqurreham me
d. Sarsam nukhai me

10. Shaqiqa ka dard kis jagha par hota hai?
a. Whole head
b. Half head
c. Kanpati me
d. Naak me

11. Daurae tamas par jazbati aur mahool ke asbab kis ke zarye ashar andaz hote hai?
a. Hypothalamus
b. Pituitary gland
c. Ovaries
d. Uterus

12. Estrogen ka ashar kis par nahi hota hai?
a. Increased vascularity of fallopian tubes
b. Pigmentation of areola
c. Breast secretion
d. Fluid secretion

13. The metabolism of progesterone occurs in:
a. Liver
b. Small intestine
c. Large intestine
d. None of the above

14. Corpus luteum ki maddat hayat kitni hai?
a. 12-14 hours
b. 24-48 hours
c. 12-14 days
d. 21 days

15. Furj ke mutaddi amraz ziyadah kab namodar hote hain?
a. During puberty
b. In reproductive life
c. Before menopause
d. After menopause

16. Which one is not found in Oral rehydration fluid?
a. Sodium chloride
b. Sodium bicarbonate
c. Potassium chloride
d. Potassium bicarbonate

17. Zaitoon ka roghan kis darakht ke seed se hasil kiya jata hai?
a. Glycine max
b. Oleo europoea

c. Acacia Arabica

d. Murr makki

18. Amale taqteer, amale tasaeed and amale takhmir ke awaleen maujood kaha ke atiba hai?

a. Unaan ke

b. Hindutan

c. Cheen

d. Arab

19. Ilmul Advia ki famous book Khazainul Advia ke musanif ka naam kiya hai?

a. Alvi kahan

b. Najmul Ghani

c. Aazam khan

d. Kabiruddin

20. Darje zail bones, carbal bone ki distal row banati hai except?

a. Trapezium

b. Triquetral

c. Trapezoid

d. Capitate

21. All of thefollowing sign and symptoms are found in Horner's syndrome except?

a. Vasoconstriction of cutaneous blod vessels of the face

b. Constricted pupil

c. Ptosis of the upper eyelid

d. Enophthalmous

22. Empty stomach ke waqt badan me kiya tabdeli hoti hai?

a. Laghri aur quwwqt me zauf

b. Farbhai aur suddo ka imkaan

c. Laghri aur suddo ka imkaan

d. Farbhai aur quwwqt me zauf

23. Sate podina ka kimiyavi naam:
a. Menthol
b. Camphor
c. Thymol
d. Oil of peppermint

24. The excess of TSH indicate:
a. Hyperthyroidism
b. Hypothyroidism
c. Simple goiter
d. Toxic goiter

25. Syndrome X ek majmavi halat hai:
a. Down syndrome
b. Klietefilters syndrome
c. Type II Diabetes mellitus
d. Diabetes insipidus

26. Secondary gout ki ek eham waja ho sakti hai:
a. Leukemia
b. Sartan-e-Kabid
c. Homocystine ki kami
d. D.M

27. Marz Pemphigus vulgaris ka taluq hai:
a. Virus se
b. Bacteria se
c. Dermatophytes
d. Autoimmune disease

28. National leprosy eradication programme kis sane isvi me shurooh hoa tha?
a. 1955
b. 1938

c. 1983

d. None of the above

29. Balon ki hifazat karne wali kaun se dawa hai?

a. Parshiyashon

b. Amla

c. Balchar

d. All of the above

30. Troponin T kis marz me investigate karte hai?

a. Cerebral Infarction

b. M.I

C. Muscular dystrophy

d. Both a & b

31. Board like rigidity is found in:

a. Diffuse peritonitis

b. Intestinal obstruction

c. Massive Ascitis

d. Intestinal T.B

32. Trendelenburg test kis joint ki stability ki janch ke liye kiya jata hai:

a. Hip joint

b. Knee joint

c. Ankle joint

d. Shoulder joint

33. Pan systolic murmur is found in:

a. M.S

b. M.R

C. A.S

d. Pulmonary valve atresia

34. Zafran kiya hai:

a. Fruit

b. Flower

c. Stigma

d. Berry

35. Ibne Sina ne Advia qalbia me kitni dawaon ka zikr hai?

a. 50

b. 63

c. 71

d. 80

36. Tap e diq ke darjat me zaboul kis darja ke liye sadir hai?

a. Darja two

b. Darja three

c. Dono Darja me

d. None of the above

37. Izme tihal ki mukhsoosh dawa hai:

a. Karanzava

b. Mako

c. Barge jhao

d. Revandchini

38. In which disease sympathectomy karte hai?

a. Buergers disease

b. Deep vein thrombosis

c. Adrenal tumor

d. Pituitary tumor

40. Which one is not cause of Coma?

a. Ketacidosis

b. Hypothermia

c. Heart failure

d. Hepatic failure

41. Jawarish shahi bilkahasoos istemal hoti hai:
a. Amraze bah me
b. Amraze meda me
c. Amraze jigar me
d. Amraze nafsani me

41. Abreham safoof karne ke liye:
a. Qainchi se bareek kaat kar garam tave par birya kar ke khural kare
b. Qainchi se kaat kar dhere dhere khural karna
c. Qainchi se kaat kar garam kar ke safoof kare
d. All of the above

42. Botanical name of Aspaghol:
a. Plantago lanta
b. Plantago ovate
c. Plantago ovait
d. Plantago menthe

43. Dejavu phenomenon is associated with:
a. Hysteria
b. Temporal lobe epilepsy
c. Melancholia
d. Anxiety neurosis

44. Habs riyah ki soorat me munasib hota hai:
a. Mulayinat ka istemal
b. Muttiyat ka istemal
c. kasir riyah ka istemal
d. Qabizat ka istemal

45. Talaiyafl kabdi ki soorat me kabid ki jasamat:
a. Big ho jati ahi
b. Small ho jati hai

c. Normal rahti hai
d. None of the above

46. Which of the following drug is not mineral origin?
a. Raskapoor
b. Mirdarsang
c. Hartal
d. Shokran

47. What are clinical features of Nephrotic syndrome?
a. Heavy proteinuria
b. Hypoproteinemia
c. Generalized edema
d. All of the above

48. Jarb-ul-Ajfan aur Damaa ke liye mufeed hai:
a. Kuhal jawahar
b. Kuhal bayaaj
c. Kuhal roshnai
d. None of the above

49. Papilledema kis marzi kaifiat me mil sakta hai?
a. Malignant hypertention
b. Diabetic retinopathy
c. Cerebral edema
d. All of the above

50. What is the length of second part of duodenum?
a. 10 cm
b. 7.5 cm
c. 2.5 cm
d. 5 cm

51. Which of the following structure is attached with Pubic Tubercle?
a. Medial end of inguinal ligament
b. Lateral end of inguinal ligament
c. Medial head of rectus abdominis
d. Lateral head of rectus abdominis

52. Lip loop ek contraceptive instrument hai jis ki jagah dosre ne lale hai:
a. Condom
b. Cu T
c. Diaphram
d. Sponge

53. Where head quarter of UNICEF is situated?
a. New York
b. Geneva
c. Washington
d. England

54. What is incubation period of Hepatitis-B?
a. 90-120 Days
b. 60-90 week
c. 60-90 Days
d. 30-60 Days

55. Functional murmur is found in:
a. Pregnancy and anemia
b. Thyrotoxicosis
c. Septal defect
d. Both a & b

56. J.V.P is raised in:
a. RHF
b. Superior vena caval obstruction
c. Tumor of upper mediastinum

d. All of the above

57. What is temperament of Mosame Rabee?
a. Har ratab
b. Barid ratab
c. Har yabis
d. Motadil

58. In which of the following the attack of Influenza is less common?
a. Children
b. Young
c. Old
d. Women's

59. When infectious agents are inters and multiply and increase their growth and number this is definition of?
a. Infection
b. Contamination
c. Infestation
d. Incubation

60. Qairooti murakkab hai:
a. Moom aur Pani
b. Moom aur Roghan
c. Roghan aur sharab
d. Roghan aur pani

61. Which of the fibrous joint?
a. Sutures
b. Symphysis
c. Hinge joint
d. Ball and socket joint

62. Tiryaq-e-Pechis kis ka murakkab hai?
a. Safoof

b. Majoon

c. Habb

d. Qurs

63. Zeeqan nafs me kaun sa mufeed murakkab hai?

a. Sharbat-e-Deenar

b. Sharbat-e-Zofa

c. Sharbat-e-Banafsha

d. Sharbat-e-Neelofar

64. The floor of Carotid triangle is made up following muscles except?

a. Superior belly of omohyoid

b. Hyoglossus

c. Thyrohyoid

d. Middle constrictor

65. Sammulfar kis me hota hai

a. Habb-e-Seen

b. Habb-e-Shifa

c. Habb-e-Qilqil

d. Habb-e-Sara

66. Deg bhabka kitne parts se bana hai?

a. 2

b. 3

c. 4

d. 5

67. Which modern instrument is used for preparation of Kushat?

a. Pulverizer

b. Autoclave

c. Muffle furnance

d. Mixer

68. What is cause of Farmers Lung?

a. Lead

b. Baggasse

c. Asbestos

d. Hay and grain dust

69. Which of the following oil is used in Juzam?

a. Olive oil

b. Turmeric oil

c. Chalmogra oil

d. Almond oil

70. Health economy is related with Unani Tibb in which manner?

a. Temperament of drugs

b. Murakkabat

c. Abdale Advia

d. Musleh

71. Kitabul nabat kis ki hai

a. Zakkaria Razi ki

b. Abu Haneefa ahmad bin Daud denouri

c. Ibne Sina

d. Ishaq bin Hannain

72.Mahloob ki istelah mustamil hai:

a. Para ke tasfia ke liye

b. Abrak ke tasfia ke liye

c. Kharateen ke tasfia ke liye

d. None of the above

73. How much time corpus luetum persist during pregnancy?

a. Upto thrre month

b. Throughout pregnancy

c. Upto 6th months
d. Upto 10th months

74. What is the commonest site of female genital cancer?
a. Cervix
b. Uterus
c. Vagina
d. Fallopian tubes

75. Myoma ki waja se aam taur par hasbe zail kaifaiat hoti hai:
a. Metorrhagia
b. Epimenorrhea
c. Haemangioma
d. Menorhhagia

76. Vitamin K ka taluq hasbe zail me se kis ki synthesis se hota hai:
a. Vitamin D
b. Coagulation factors
c. Both a & b
d. None

77. Congenital Tuberculosis baccho me kis tarah se shurooh ho sakta hai?
a. Transplacental infection
b. Amniotic fluid
c. Amniocentesis
d. None of them

78. What is the head circumference of child during birth?
a. 40 cm
b. 30 cm
c. 50 cm

d. 35 cm

79. Symphysis pubis ki Nichli satah par urethra kis zarye attached hota hai?
a. Pubocervical ligament
b. Transverse cervical ligament
c. Suspensory ligament
d. None of the above

80. Skenes glands are homologous to:
a. Testes in male
b. Scrotum in male
c. Prostate in male
d. None of the above

81. What is other name of Mackenrodts Ligament?
a. Round ligament
b. Broad ligament
c. Ovarian ligament
d. Cardinal ligament

82. Alpha and Beta, adrenergic and cholinergic receptors kaha hote hain?
a. Myometrium
b. Parametrium
c. Endometrium
d. None of the above

83. Amal e Tayir kiya hai:
a. Furzaja
b. Huqna
c. Hamool
d. Nafookh

84. Which sakht is passed deep to hypoglossus?
a. Facial artery

b. Lingual nerve

c. Lingual artery

d. Nerve to mylohyoid

85. Cervical plexus se darje zail shakhai nikalti hai except?

a. Mucular branches to sternocleidomastoid

b. Phrenic nerve

c. Descendens hypoglossi

d. Mucular branches to prevertibral muscles

86. Raskapoor ek murakkab hai:

a. Phitkari and gile Armani ka

b. Semaab aur Shibbe yamani ka

c. Semaab, phitkari and gile Armani

d. None of the above

87. Which of the following is not an example of Synovial joints?

a. Hinge

b. Syndesmosis

c. Pivot

d. Saddle

88. Kis ka nafa khas taqwiyate jigar hai:

a. Majoon-e-Aqrab

b. Majoon-e-Kabir

c. Majoon-e-Dabidulwarad

d. Majoon-e-Injabar

89. Ma jaiudul-johar ka zariya kaun sa pani hai?

a. Chashmon ka paani

b. Barish ka paani

c. Kuano ka paani

d. Nallo ka paani

90. Jawarish kamooni ka main ingredient hai:
a. Bahidana
b. Filfil siyah
c. Zeera siyah
d. Zanjabeel

91. Klumpkes palsy me kaun sa lesion mutashir hota hai?
a. C5, C6, C7
b. C5, C6
c. C8, T1
d. C4, C5, C6

92.Facial nerve ki motor root darje zail tamaam azlaat ki asabi parvarish karate hai except?
a. Muscles of facial expression
b. Platysma
c. Posterior belly of diagastric
d. Masseter

93. Lauq katan ki tarkeeb me shamil kiya jata hai:
a. Luab tukhm katan
b. Tukhm katan
c. Safoof tukhm katan
d. Barg katan

94. Wrist drop is caused due to injury of which nerve?
a. Ulnar
b. Radial
c. Median
d. Musculocutaneous

95. Oculomotor nerve ki injury ya division se upper lid ki drooping kis azla ki paralysis ki waja se paida hoti hai?
a. Superior rectus

b. Inferior rectus

c. Levator Palpabre superioris

d. Inferior rectus

96. Qiwam banate waqt jhaag utar kar mail saaf karne kea mal ko kiya kahte hai?

a. Isnan

b. Tasfia

c. Ahraque

d. Irgha

97. Spinal cord, vertebra ke kis level par end hoti hai?

a. Lower border of L2

b. Upper border of L3

c. Lower border of L1

d. Upper border of L1

98. Quwwate moalida aur masowira se murakkab hai:

a. Qwwatwe Hawania

b. Nafsania

b. Tanasulia

d. None of the above

99. Length of Prostatic urethra is:

a. 3 cm

b. 4 cm

c. 10 cm

d. 20 cm

100. Adductor canal ke darje zail mashmolaat hain except?

a. Femoral artery

b. Femoral artey

c. Saphenous artery

d. Adductor magnus

101. Where the training and research centre for Filaria is situated?
a. Koze coat (Kali cut)
b. Raja mandarin
c. Banaras
d. All of the above

102. Following are the methods for control of reservoir except?
a. Early diagnosis
b. Notification
c. Treatment
d. Active immunizarion

103. Human herpese virus-3 is cause of which disease?
a. Small pox
b. Chicken pox
c. Measles
d. Mumps

104. Loss of pubic hair, axillary hair, secondary amenorrhea and atrophy of breasts kis syndrome ki alaamat hai?
a. Turners syndrome
b. Stein-leveithal syndrome
c. Ashermans syndrome
d. Sheehans syndrome

105. Full term nauzaidh bchcho me Physiological jaundice ka incidence kitne percentage hai?
a. 20-30%
b. 30-40%
c. 40-50%
d. 50-60%

106. Night blindness is caused by deficiency of:
a. Vitamin-D
b. Vitamin-B12
c. Vitamin-A
d. Vitamin-C

107. What is colur of stool in Cholera?
a. Yellowish colour
b. White colour
c. Siyah colour
d. Surkhi colour

108. Zaheer amoebai ek:
a. Metabolic disease
b. Infectious disease
c.. Neurotic disease
d. Congestive disease

109. What is length of small intestine is?
a. 3meters
b. 5meters
c. 6.5meters
d. 9meters

110. Cause of headache is Tafarruke ittesal, this statement was given by:
a. Jalinoos
b. Ibne Sina
c. Arasto
d. None of the above

111. Sehat wa marz me malka adam malka ka taaluq hai:
a. Jalinoos ke nazdeek
b. Ibne Sina ke nazdeek
c. Done ke nazdeek

d. None of the above

112. Net maternal weight gain kitna hota hai?
a. 12 kg
b. 10 kg
c. 8 kg
d. 6 kg

113. Marz Zatul janab me:
a. Lungs sukar jate hai
b. Mutwarrim ho jate hai
c. Ghishurriya mutwarrim ho jati hai
d. Ghishurriya ke ander hawa ikattha ho jati hai

114. Placenta ke main functions hasbe zail hote hai except?
a. Oxygnation
b. Respiratory
c. Excretory
d. Nuttritory

115. Placental sepration kis hisse se hota hai?
a. Decidua basalis
b. Decidua Capsularis
c. Decidua Spongiosum
d. None of the above

116. Shakar Tighal ka makhiz hai:
a. Nabati
b. Haiwani
c. Jamadati
d. Masnawi

117. Boul-e-Kurrasi qism hai:
a. Boul-e-Ahmar ki
b. Boul-e-Akhzar ki

c. Boul-e-Asfar ki
d. Boul-e-Aswad ki

118. Retinol (Vitamin A) daje zail me sabse ziyadah paya jata hai:
a. Liver oil
b. Carrot oil
c. Margraine
d. Butter

119. Hindustani ghiza ke total enegy intake me protein ka daje zail fesad taun hai:
a. 65-80 %
b. 15-30 %
c. 7-15 %
d.1-7 %

120. Boul-e-Tabni dalalat karta hai:
a. Mizaj ke barodat ki
b. Kasrate mayiyat ki
c. Qilate safra ki
d. All of the above

121. Fauri tadbeer naumolood (early neonatal care) me darj zaroori nahi hai:
a. Afale qalb wa tanafus ko qaim karna
b. Jism ki hararat ko qaim karna
c. Wazan ko qaim karna
d. Infection se bacchna

122. Istisqa mishal hai:
a. Wame damwi
b. Wame Balghamii
c. Wame Mayi
d. Wame Rehi

123. Mandarja zail ehtabas ghair tabai ka sabab nahi hai:

a. Quwwate masika quwwa ho jai

b. Quwwate hazima zaeef ho jai

c. Quwwate tabiya dosree taraf muwaje ho jai

d. Quwwate dafia kam ho jai

124. All are granulomatous diseases except?

a. TB

b. Leprosy

c. Sarcoidosis

d. Amoebiasis

125. Leucocytosis is not seen:

a. Typhoid

b. MI

c. Appendicitis

d. Measles

126. BCG Vaccine is:

a. Live attenuated

b. Killed/Inactivated

c. Toxoid

d. Combined

127. Mubaridat ke asbab ho sakte hai:

a. Ehtabas wa istefragh ki ziyadti

b. Sukoon wa neend ki ziyadti

c. Barid makolat wa Mashrobat ka istemal

d. All of the above

128. Second trimester me abortion ki sab se aham wajah kiya hai?

a. Cervical uterine factor

b. Endocervical factor

c. Both a & b

d. None

129. The most common termination of lobar pneumonia is:
a. Consolidation
b. Resolution
c. Abscess formation
d. Empyema

130. Tafarukue ittesal ka sabab ho sakta hai:
a. Khilte akaal
b. Khilte Muhariq
c. Khilte Murkhi
d. All

131. Amraze saudawi ke muaalija me mustamil hai:
a. Khameera Abresham
b. Khameera Khashkhash
c. Majoon Najah
d. Majoon ushbah

132. Ustokhuddos ka istemal mufeed hai:
a. Sar dard me
b. Kaan dard me
c. Iltihabe tajaveef aaf
d. Warmw ghishaul anaf

133.Nakho ke natejah me nawaat me paya ja sakta hai:
a. Pyknosis
b. Karyorrhexis
c. Both of the above
d. None

134. Wah asbab jin ke door ho jane ke baujood un ke asarat baki rahte hain:
a. Asbabe Mughaira

b. Asbabe Sabiqa
c. Asbabe Mukhalfa
d. Asbabe Badiah

135. Kaun si dawa Munshi hai?
a. Bazarulbanj
b. Ajwain
c. Zeerah
d. Baboona

136. Khar khusk ka mutradif naam hai:
a. Gokhro
b. Zaro
c. Khanjak
d. All of the above

137. Fadagh tafarruke ittesal hai:
a. Jild ka
b. Bone ka
c. Aasab ka
d. Azla ka

138. Pure honey me sab se ziyadah miqdar me kiya hota hai?
a. Inverted sugar
b. Dextrin
c. Sucrose
d. Wax

139. Marz khilqat qism hai:
a. Sue tarkeeb
b. Tafarruke ittesal
c. Marz adad
d. Marz wazaa ki

140. USG me Embryonic movement kab visible hote hai?

a. 6th week

b. 10th week

c. 5th week

d. 8th week

141. Fatty necrosis is found in:

a. Breast

b. Omentum

c. Both

d. None

142. Rh Anti D Immunoglobulin, mother kis waqt intramuscular dete hai?

a. After child birth

b. After abortion

c. Both of them

d. None of them

143. Revised national Tuberculosis Programme me darje zail nukta shamil hai:

a. Teeka

b. Shifa ki dar 85%

c. Balgham ka umtihaan 70%

d. DOTS

144. Primary internal piles ki darje zail positions hoti hai except?

a. 3 O clock

b. 11 O clock

c. 7 O clock

d. 9 O clock

145. In adult erythropoiesis occur in:

a. RBC

b. Bone marrow

c. WBC
d. All of them

146. The cause of smell in gangrene:
a. Ammonia
b. Indole
c. Skatole
d. All of the above

147. Qurse mussalas ka main ingredients hai:
a. Zafran
b. Afyun
c. Dhaura
d. None of the above

148. Dayaqoozah ka istemaal kiya jata hai:
a. Amraze meda
b. Amraze tanafus
c. Amraze jigar
d. Amraze aasab

149. Bhang ko mudabbar karte hai:
a. Aabe ajwain me
b. Aabe zeera siyah me
c. Aabe qinnab me
d. Aabe dhatura me

150. Rovsings sign is seen in:
a. Acute appendicitis
b. Acute cholecystitis
c. Pancreatitis
d. Parotiditis

151. Umblical cord descent ke kitne types hote hai?
a. Cord presentation
b. Cord prolapsed

c. Occult prolapsed
d. All of them

152. Uzue rais sirf dimagh hai:
a. Ye khayal- Buqraat ka
b. Ye khayal- Ibne Sina ka
c. Ye khayal- Jalinoos ka
d. Ye khayal- Razi ka

153. Qutube shumali kahte hai:
a. Rabai maskoon ka doosra naam hai
b. Pahli aqleem ko
c. Second aqleem ko
d. Seventh aqleem ko

154. The cause of death in acute inversion of uterus is:
a. Shock
b. Hemorrhage
c. Embolism
d. All of the above

155. The gas used for analgesia is:
a. Oxygen
b. Nitrous oxide
c. Co2
d. None of the above

156. Aazai asaliya kahte hain:
a. Azai murakkaba
b. Azai mufrada
c. Azai mutshabatul aaza ko
d. None of the above

157. What is infancy?
a. First month of life
b. First year of life

c. Second year of life

d. Second month of life

158. Antihypertensive treatment of a patient is:

a. Stopped a day before operation

b. Stopped a week before operation

c. Stopped two days before operation

d. Continued till the date of operation

159. Boule Fuqaai is a type of:

a. Boule ahmar

b. Boule akhzar

c. Boule aswad

d. Boule abiyaz

160. Fatty infiltration me shaham ko rang sakte hai:

a. H & E stain se

b. Sudan III se

c. Both of them

d. None of them

161. Which of the following drug is hepatotoxic?

a. Ketamine

b. Thiopentone

c. Halothane

d. None of the above

162. Mizaj-e- Motadil tareen kahlata hai:

a. Mizaj-e-Aqaleem

b. Mizaj-e-Nabati

c. Mizaj-e-Insaani

d. None of the above

163. Which of the following is not a volatile anesthetic agent?

a. Ether

b. Halothane

c. Isoflurane

d. Propofol

164. Ifadah kabir mujmil hai:

a. Alqanoon ka khulasa

b. Sharah asbab ka khulasa

c. Dono ka khulasa

d. Kisi ka nahi

165. Tamaam aaza me sab se ziyadah motadil shadat ki ungli hai ye khayal hai:

a. Ibne Sina ka

b. Jalinoos ka

c. Buqrat ka

d. None of the above

166. Laryngoscopy and tracheal intubation may give rise to:

a. Increase in heart

b. Increase blood pressure

c. Cardiac arrhythmias

d. All of the above

167. In portal hypertension the sites of portosystemic anastomosis are:

a. Lower end of oesophagus

b. Around umbilicus

c. Lower third of rectum and anal canal

d. All of the above

168. Seminoma testis is:

a. Seen in very old patient

b. Always bilateral

c. Seen in patients above thirty years of age

d. A benign tumor

169. Kushta Tootia ka fail hai:
a. Muqawwi-e-Asab
b. Dafa-e-Atishk
c. Muddamil qarooh
d. All of the above

170. Bony metastasis in carcinoma of prostate appear as:
a. Soup bubble appearance
b. Osteolytic area
c. Osteoblastic area
d. Sunray appearance

171. Wilms tumor occurs in the age group of:
a. 2 to 5 years
b, 12 to 15 years
c. 20 to 30 years
d. 40 to 60 years

172. Canograph shows the concentration of:
a. N_2O
b. O_2
c. H_2
d. CO_2

173. Carpel tunnel syndrome me mutashirah nerve hai:
a. Median nerve
b. Ulnar nerve
c. Radial nerve
d. Popleteal nerve

174. In upper GI Endoscopy the stomach is distended with:
a. CO_2
b. N2o

c. Normal air

d. Ammonia

175. The chances of Liver malignancy are more in patient who have had?

a. Hepatitis A

b. Hepatitis B

c. Hepatitis E

d. Amoebic Hepatitis

176. Cullens sign is seen in:

a. Acute cholecystitis

b. Acute appendicitis

c. Acute hemorrhagic pancreatitis

d. Acute Gastritis

177. Potts puffy tumor is:

a. A benign tumor of testis

b. A malignant tumor

c. An infective condition of scalp

d. An infective condition of spine

178. All predispose to oral cancer except?

a. Erytroplakia

b. Leukoplakia

c. Submucous fibrosis

d. Oral lichenplanus

179. Mannitol is usedin all except?

a. Tumorogenic oedema

b. Vasculogenic edema

c. Hepatic encephalopathy

d. Intracranial hemorrhage

180. Barrets ulcer is due to?

a. Ischaemia

b. Ectopic gastric mucosa

c. Bile reflux

d. Reflux esophagitis

181. The courvoisiers law is related to:

a. Fistula in ano

b. Jaundice

c. Portal hypertension

d. Carcinoma stomach

182. Dielts crisis is seen in:

a. Renal cell carcinoma

b. Hydronephrosis

c. Hemorrhagic shock

d. After thyroid surgery

183. Urinary bladder tumor mostly arises from:

a. Mucosa

b. Submucosa

c. Muscle layer

d. Serosa

184. Pulsating varicose vein in young adult is due to:

a. Arteriovenus fistula

b. Saphenofemoral incompitance

c. Deep vein thrombosis

d. Abdominal tumor

185. The commonest cause of benign surgical jaundice is:

a. CBD stone

b. CBD stricture

c. Carcinoma pancreas

d. Carcinoma of gall bladder

186. Incompletely descended testis is most common on:
a. Right side
b. Both sides
c. Left side
d. None of the above

187. Which of the following parts of body is not affected by leprosy?
a. Testis
b. Ovary
c. Nasal mucosa
d. Axilla

188. Urine karte waqt bladder ka pressure kitna hota hai:
a. 35-50 cm H2O
b. 20-25 cm H2O
c. 35-50 mmHg
d. 100-150 mmHg

189. Tetany hone ke liye Serum calcium ka kam hona:
a. Zaroori hai
b. Normal serum calcium me bhi ho sakta hai
c. Ziyadah serum calcium me bhi ho sakti hai
d. None of the above

190. What is primary hemorrhage?
a. Blood loss during operation
b. After opration
c. At the site of operation
d. None of the above

191. What is Clostridium tetani?
a. Gram positive Rods
b. Gram negative Rods
c. AFB Rods

d. Gram positive Spore

192. Adenoma kis tissue ka tumor hai?
a. Secretary gland ka
b. Connective tissue ka
c. Muscle tissue ka
d. None of the above

193. Plexiform neurofibromatosis kis nerve ke saath hita hai?
a. IV nerve
b. V Cranial nerve
c. Peripheral nerve
d. VI cranial neve

194. Claudication distance ko kis tarah se define karte hai?
a. Dard se pahle ki doori
b. Clot banne se pahle ki doori
c. None of the above
d. Both a and b

195. Dermoid cyst mandarja zail me se kiya haia?
a. Acquired cyst
b. Developmental cyst
c. Implanted cyst
d. Retension cyst

196. Salivary glands me sab se ziyadah tumor kaun se gland me hota hai?
a. Parotid gland
b. Submandibular gland
c. Sublingual gland
d. None of the above

197. Hernia ke content me kaun se cheez hoti hai jab is ko Richters herni kahte hai?

a. Omentum

b. Bowel loop

c. Appendix

d. Circumference of bowel

198. Arqe kasni kasheed kiya jata hai:

a. Gule kasni se

b. Tukhm kasni se

c. Barg kasni se

d. Beikh kasni se

199. Rooh tahallul barh jata ahi:

a. Khushi me

b. Fasad me

c. Jamaa me

d. All of the above

200. Filfil daraz ka nabati naam mandarja zail me se kiya hai?

a. Piper longum

b. Piper nigrum

c. Piper cubeba

d. Piper betel

MD AMU ENTRANCE EXAMNATION
ANSWERS KEY 2010-11

1. B   2. A   3. A   4. C   5. A
6. B   7. B   8. A   9. D   10. B
11. A   12. C   13. A 14. C   15. D
16. D   17. B   18. D   19. B   20. B
21. A   22. A   23. A   24. B   25. C
26. A   27. D   28. C   29. D   30. B
31. A   32. A   33. B   34. C   35. B
36. A   37. C   38. A   39. C   40. D
41. A   42. B   43. B   44. C   45. B
46. D   47. D   48. A   49. D   50. B
51. A   52. B   53. A   54. C   55. D
56. D   57. D   58. A   59. A   60. B
61. A   62. A   63. B   64. A   65. A
66. C   67. C   68. D   69. C   70. C
71. B   72. B   73. B   74. A   75. D
76. B   77. A   78. D   79. C   80. C
81. D   82. A   83. B   84. C   85. A
86. C   87. B   88. C   89. A   90. C
91. C   92. D   93. A   94. B   95. C
96. D   97. C   98. C   99. A   100.D
101.D   102.D   103.B   104.D 105.D
106.C   107.B   108.B   109.C   110.A
111.B   112.D   113.C   114.A   115.A
116.B   117.B 118.A   119.C   120.D
121.C   122.C   123.D   124.D   125.A
126.A   127.D   128.A   129.B   130.D
131.C   132.C   133.C   134.C   135.A
136.D   137.D   138.A   139.A   140.D
141.C   142.C   143.A 144.D   145.B
146.D   147.B   148.B   149.A   150.A
151.D   152.A   153.D   154.D   155.B
156.B 157.B   158.D   159.D   160.B
161.C   162.C   163.D   164.A   165.B

166.D 167.D 168.C 169.D 170.C
171.A 172.D 173.A 174.C 175.B
176.C 177.C 178.C 179.D 180.B
181.B 182.B 183.A 184.A 185.A
186.A 187.B 188.A 189.B 190.A
191.A 192.A 193.B 194.A 195.B
196.A 197.D 198.C 199.D 200.A

1. Aqleem Rabai kis khate arz ke qareeb hai?

a. Khate istiwa

b. Khate sartan

c. Khate jiddi

d. Qutube sumali

2. Kitabul asbab wa al alamaat likhi hai:

a. Najeebuddin Samarqandi ne

b. Hakeem khuwajah Rizwan ahmad ne

c. Hakeem kabiruddin ne

d. Hakeem sharif kahan ne

3. Safara kin aaza ke taghzia me shamil hai?

a. Lungs

b. Cartilage

c. B.V

d. All of the above

4. Sharaiyn ugti hain qalb se vareedai ugti hain jigar se ye qaul kis ka hai?

a. Buqrat ka

b. Aflatoon ka

c. Ibne Sina ka

d. Jalinoos ka

5. Quwwate mufakkarah, mutakhaila aur Hafiza se anjam pata hai:

a. Taghzia

b. Tanqia

c. Hazm

d. None of the above

6. Akhlat me nuzaj paida hota hai:
a. Meda me
b. Jigar me
c. Spleen me
d. Pancreas me

7. Hararate gharizi ki ibtida hoti hai:
a. Maa ke stomach se
b. At the time of birth
c. Both of the above
d. None of the above

8. Quwwate mudraka hai:
a. Quwwate Haiwania ka part
b. Quwwate Tabaiyah ka part
c. Quwwate Nafsania ka part
d. None of the above

9. Mizaj motadil tibbi bana hai:
a. Adal fil Qismat se
b. Barabar taqseem se
c. Both of the above
d. None of the above

10. Aazai Haiwamia me shamil hai:
a. Qalb
b. Jigar
c. Dimagh
d. None of the above

11. Quwwat e ghaziah ka fail hai:
a. Taghzia ko rokna
b. Taghzia ko anjam dena
c. Both of the above
d. None of the above

12. Khoon ka mazah hai:
a. Malah
b. Hamiz
c. Affis
d. None of the above

13. Teen anasir ke nazariyah me kaun se anasir shamil hai:
a. Hawa, Naar. Arz
b. Malah, duhan, kibriyat
c. Malah, parah, kibriyat
d. None of the above

14. Anasir naar ka tabai muqaam:
a. Kurrah-e-Arz ke bad
b. Kurrah-e-Maa se pahle
c. Kurrah-e-Maa ke bad
d. Kurrah-e-Hawa ke bad

15. Emam Fakhruddin Razi ke mutabiq motadil tareen aqleem kaun se hai:
a. Aqleem first
b. Aqleem second
c. Aqleem third
d. Aqleem fourth

16. Balgham Hamiz ka Mizaj:
a. Sarde wa khushki ki taraf mail hota hai
b. Sarde wa taree ki taraf mail hota hai
c. Har ratab hota hai
d. None of the above

17. Mirrah safra wah safra hai jis ke sath:
a. Balgham Ghaliz mil jai
b. Balgham Raqeeq mil jai
c. Balgham Yabis mil jai

d. None of the above

18. Kitabul kuliyat kis musanif ki Takhleeq hai?
a. Ibne Rushd
b. Kamaluddin Hussain Hamdaani
c. Abusahal Masihi
d. Saikh Ibne Sina

19. Mizaj motadil Shakhsi bilqiyas ilal kharij kis ki qism hai?
a. Mizaj motadil Tibbi
b. Mizaj motadil Ghair Tibbi
c. Mizaj motadil Shakhsi
d. Sue Mizaj Shakhsi

20. Bareetoon kis ki mishal hai?
a. Ghishai rabati ki
b. Ghishai safaqi ki
c. Ghishai maai ki
d. Ghishai mufasali ki

21. Ratoobate azali kaha payi jati hai?
a. Laham gudoodi
b. Laham khusaiyatain
c. Laham saddaiyai
d. None of the above

22. Quwwate Tabayia me kaun se quwwatain shamil hain?
a. Quwwate shakhsia, Quwwate munfaila
b. Quwwate faila, Quwwate tanasulia
c. Quwwate ghazia Quwwate jaziba
d. None of theaboove

23. Sabhi gram munshibit jarashim hain except?
a. Streptococci

b. Staphylococci
c. Meningococci
d. Pneumococci

24. Falghamooni kahte hai:
a. Warme Damwi ko
b. Warme Safrawi ko
c. Warme Balghami ko
d. None of the above

25. Jism me musakhinat ka sabab ho sakta hai:
a. Motadil moqdaar me ghiza ka istemaal
b. Motadil moqdaar ki harakat
c. Ufoonat ka hona
d. All of the above

26. Judri mishaal hai:
a. Bushoore damwi
b. Bushoore safrawi
c. Bushoore saudawi
d. Bushoore balghami

27. Ittesai majari ka sabab hai:
a. Quwwate masika ka zaeef hona
b. Advia mushila ka istemaal
c. Advia murkhiaa ka istemaal
d. All of the above

28. Liquefactive necrosis is found in:
a. Brain
b. Liver
c. Heart
d. Spleen

29. Nafakh mishaal hai:
a. Warme har ki

b. Warme barid ki
c. Warme maai ki
d. Warme reehi ki

30. Kuriyate hamara ka Qatr mutfaraq hota hai:
a. Poikilocytosis
b. Anisocytosis
c. Microcytosis
d. Macrocytosis

31. Juzam ke jarasheem ko rangane ke liye istemaal karte hai:
a. Grams stain
b. Ziel Neelsens stain
c. Leishmans stain
d. Geimsa stain

32. Pseudomembranous inflammation paya jata hai:
a. Tonsilitis
b. Pharyngitis
c. Diphtheria
d. Laryngitis

33. Boule naari qism hai hai:
a. Boule asfar
b. Boule ahmar
c. Boule akhzar
d. Boule aswad

34. Zarqah kis uzu ka marz hai?
a. Ear
b. Eye
c. Nail
d. Jild

35. Mufattah Shaab Advia se kis cheez me izafa ho jata hai?
a. Total lung capacity me
b. Vital capacity me
c. Khoon ke under O2 ki kimmiyat
d. All of the above

36. Zingari balgham kharij hota hai:
a. Shaheeqa me
b. Taqeehul sadar me
c. Zatur riya me
d. Nafakhatur riya me

37. Ittesai qalb ki soorat me:
a. Qalb me waram lahiq ho jata hai
b. Qalb ke batan dialate ho jate hai
c. Qalb ke batan narrow ho jate hai
d. Azlate qalb me motapa ho jata hai

38. Arrhytmia ki aham wajah ho sakti hai:
a. K+ ki kami and Mg++ ki kami
b. Na+ ki kami and K+ ki ziyadti
c. K+ ki ziyadti and Na+ ki ziyadti
d. Mg++ ki ziyadti and K+ ki kami

39. Rheumatic heart disease ke liye Jones Major Criteria me kiya shamil nahi hai?
a. Carditis
b. Subcutaneous nodoule
c. Fever
d. Chorea

40. Deedane jarb hote hain:
A. Bacteria
b. Virus
c. Fungus

d. Mites

41. Apple gelly appearance kis jildi marz me dekhne ko milte hai?
a. Jild ki tuberculosis me
b. Pemphigus
c. Jild ke sartan me
d. Bahaq abiyaz me

42. Basoore labaniya ka aham sabab kiya hai?
a. Shami madde ka kasrat afaraz
b. Fasade balgham
c. Tadiya
d. Safra ka ghalba

43. Austiz sign kis bemari ka sign hai?
a. Quba
b. Hikkah
c. Psoriosis
d. Shara

44. Maqad me jamma karane ki shaded khwahish ko kahte hain:
a. Aqoona
b. Ubna
c. Azyoot
d. Elaous

45. Gurdon ki pathri ka faili sabab:
a. Hararat hai
b. Barodat hai
c. Ghaliz lesdar ratoobat
d. Ghurdah ka zaeef hona

46. Khuwahish jamaa quwwa ho jati hai:
a. Sue mizaj gurdah har me

b. Sue mizaj gurdah barid me

c. Both a and b

d. None of the above

47. Plague ka makhsoos Jarshoma kiya hai:

a. Yersinia pestis

b. Flavi virus

c. Para myxovirus

d. Shigella bacilli

48. Marz Juzam paida hota hai hai:

a. Dam mohtaraq ke badan me phail jane ke bass

b. Balghab zujaji ke badan me phail jane ke bass

c. Safra ghaliz ke badan me phail jane ke bass

d. Mirrah sauda ke badan me phail jane ke bass

49. Miayadi bukahar me first week me Positive hota hai:

a. Widal test

b. Blood test

c. Urine test

d. Stool test

50. Safoof Muqlisha khas taur par mufeed hai:

a. Yarqan me

b. Jaul Baqar

c. Zaheer muzmin

d. Nazla muzmin

51. Qoolanj Rasasi hota hai:

a. Dedane Aama ki waja

b. Basoor Aama ki waja

c. Seesa ki simiyat ki waja

d .Qabz ki waja

52. Taqhaqar mari wa meda ziyadah paya jata hai:
a. In old
b. In children
c. Sheer khuar baccho me
d. Nasha karne walon me

53. Helicobater is cause of:
a. Cancer of stomach
b. Ulcer of stomach
c. Duodenal ulcer
d. All of the above

54.Commonest site of cancer in stomach:
a. Pyloric part
b. Cardiac part
c. Greater curvature
d. All of the above

55. The complication of Hepatitis B is:
a. Saqoote qalb
b. Talayaful kabid
c. Sartane kabid
d. All of the above

56. Alzheimers disease ki sab se aham alamat hai:
a. Quwwat gauhai ka foat ho jana
b. Quwwat fiqr me fasad ka lahiq ho jana
c. Azlaat me jamood ka paida ho jana
d. Nisyaan ka paida ho jana

57. Sudaee khumari me sar me dard kab ariz hota hai:
a. Galiz aur kuhna sharab se
b. Sar me chhot lagne se
c. Bukharat ke dimagh ki taraf saood karne se
d. Fsad akhlat se

58. Marz junoon:
a. Fasid Balgham se paida hota hai
b. Fasid Safara se paida hota hai
c. Fasid Dam se paida hota hai
d. Fasid Sauda se paida hota hai

59. Majoon lina mufeed hai:
a. Zaufe Aasab me
b. Zaufe Qalb me
c. Zaufe Hazam me
d. Zaufe Kuliya me

60. Mazoorat se murad hain wah basoor jo taiyar kiye jate hain:
a. Gaust ke sath
b. Bones ke sath
c. Vegatables ke sath
d. None of the above

61. Musammin, Murghan, Muqawwi wa kaseer miqdaar me ghizai ilaj hai:
a. Sartan ka
b. Diq ka
c. Jiyaan ka
d. Kasrate tams ka

62. Istifragh bila nujiz kis halat me karaya ja sakta hai?
a. Jab madda me hejan ho
b. Jab madda doosri janib muntaqil ho raha ho
c. Amraze hada me
d. All of the above

63. Saddle back type of temperature is found in:
a. Brucellosis
b. Dengue fever
c. Viral fever

d. Enteric fever

64. Hummiyate ufoonia me kis cheez ka istemal har waqt kiya ja sakta hai?
a. Sikanjabeen ka
b. Fawakihat ka
c. Mubarridat ka
d. Mushilat ka

65. Lifooria kahte hain us bukhar ko jis me:
a. Badan ke ander ghair mamoolii hararat aur bahar sardi maaloom hoti ho
b. Badan ke ander baroodat aur bahar hararat maaloom hoti ho
c. Badan ke ander aur bahar ghair mamoolii hararat
d. Badan ke ander aur bahar khafeef hararat

66. Which lipid increase during exercise?
a. Triglyceride
b. HDL
c. LDL
d. All of the above

67. Hakeem Akbar Arzani ka tarteeb diya hoa Sharbat:
a. Sharbate Ahmad Shahi
b. Sharbate Firya daras
c. Sharbate Ezaj
d. Sharbate Rabvi

68. Israrul adviatul murakkaba ka musanif hai:
a. Hanain ibne Ishaaq
b. Abu nasar attar israili
c. Uhina bin Maswia
d. Najeebuddin Samar qandi

69. Asbabul nabataat ka musanif hai:

a. Desiqurdoos

b. Saufrastus

c. Feeshaghauras

d. Ibne Hubbal

70. Dawa sazi ki mashhoor tareen kitab Minhajul Dukkan wa dustoorul Ayyan fi tarkeebul Advia ka musanif hai:

a. Abunasar jalali

b. Abul QASIM Farishta

c. Abu Reehan Albeerooni

d. Abu Nasar attar

71. Simaab ko jism se nikalne ke liye istemaal karte hai:

a. Pettha

b. Leemo kaghzi

c. Madar ki lakri ka koyla

d. All of the above

72. Kavi dawa ka istemal hota hai:

a. Rasooli ki tahleel

b. Iltihabe muzmin ki tahleel

c. Sharyain ke Habs dam ke liye

d. All of the above

73. Mushil bil talayyan hai:

a. Turbud

b. Sheer khasht

c. Resha khatmi

d. Saqmonia

74. Kisi dawa ka half life ziyadah hai to:

a. Is ka duration action kam hoga

b. Is ka duration action Ziyadah hoga

c. Is ki efficacy ziyadah hogi

d. Is ki efficacy kam hogi

75. The route in which bioavailability of drug is 100%?
a. Oral
b. Through anus
c. Injection
d. None of the above

76. Kushta sazi ke hawale se darjate hararat ko:
a. 2 Darjat me taqsim kiya gyaa hai
b. 3 Darjat me taqsim kiya gyaa hai
c. 4 Darjat me taqsim kiya gyaa hai
d. 5 Darjat me taqsim kiya gyaa hai

77. Majoon Zabeeb ka nafa khas hai:
a. Nafa Shara
b. Muharik Bah
c. Muqawwi meda
d. Muqawwi aza raisa

78. Kushta abrak safed mustamil hai hai:
a. Seelanurreham
b. Sual me
c. Jiryaan me
d. All of the above

79. Tiryaqe pechis ka main ingredient hai:
a.Amla munaqa
b. Tukhm Haloon
c. Haleela zarad
d. Haleela siyah

80. Al-ahmar tayyar kiya jata hai:
a. Shangaraf + Mettha teliya
b. Sammulfar + Beesh ke satth
c. Shangaraf + Jadwar ke satth

d. Shangaraf + Sammulfar+ Hartal tabki ke satth

81. Kushta Gaudanti mustamil hai hai:
a. Humme tifoodiya
b. Humme mevia
c. Zeeqanaffas sabaai
d. Humme ijamia

82. Marham risl ka main ingredient hai:
a. Tootiya
b. Raal
c. Gandah bahrozah
d. Mirdaar sang

83. Ajazai lateefa hasil karte hain bazrya:
a. Jarulqi
b. Amale taqsheer
c. Amale takes
d. Amale Tabloor

84. Johare seen hasil karte hai bazarye:
a. Amale tadkheen
b. Amale tadheen
c. Amale tareeque
d. Amale taseed

85. Amale tarweeq kis dawa ke kiye makhsoos hai:
a. Barge chiraita sabz wa saatar farsi sabz
b. Tukhm mako wa tukhm kasni
c. Barg mako sabz wa barg kasni sabz
d. Barg kasundhi sabz wa barg katail sabz

86. Unani murakkabat me qurs banana ke liye kis binder ka istemaal sab se ziyadah hota hai?
a. Muqil
b. Samagh arabi

c. Luaab

d. Kundur

87. Zingaar ka chemical name:

a. Copper sulphate

b. Copper oxide

c. Copper disulphate

d. Zinc sulphate

88. Sange jarahat ka chemical name:

a. Magnesium trisilicate

b. Hydrated Magnesium silicate

c. Potassium oxide

d. Aluminium hydraoxide

89. Musakin alam wa muzafif ratoobaat afal hamil dawa ka naam hai:

a. Ajwain khurasani

b. Ajwain desi

c. Podeena

d. Ajmoad

90. Sareesham mahi bilkhasoos mustamil hai:

a. Nafsuddam

b. Nakseer

c. Zeeqannafas shabaai

d. Suale nazalawi

91. Kunjad ka kaun hissa dawa me istemaal hita hai:

a. Root

b. Leaves

c. Seed and oil

d. Ratoobat

92. Mazo sabz kiya hai?

a. Ek podhe ka phal hai

b. Ek keerae ka ghar hai

c. Ek madani dawa hai

d. Ek podhe ki kali hai

93. Aatrilal belongs which family?

a. Apiaceae

b. Fagaceae

c. Solanaceae

d. Astraceae

94. Kisi bhi alkaloid me carbon, hydrogen and oxygen ke alavah kis dosre unsure ka hona lazmi hai?

a. Sulphur

b. Bromine

c. Chlorine

d. Nitrogen

95. Filfil safed kis tarah hasil karte hota hai:

a. Filfil siyah ko multaani me dibo kar khusk kar lete hai

b. Dono alag alag podho se hasil hota hai

c. Filfil siyah ke oopri kali satah (Epicorp) ko nikal kar hasil karte hai

d. Filfil siyah ke kachche phal ko filfil safed kahte hai

96. Shangaraf hasbe zail me se kis unsoor ka salt hai?

a. Hg

b. Pb

c. As

d. Cu

97. Corylus avellana ka Unani name kiya hai?

a. Fandaq

b. Sammulfar

c. Suddab

d. Todri

98. Joz Mashal ka nabati name hasbe zail me se kaun sa hai:
a. Datura stramonium
b. Hyosyamus niger
c. Myristic fragrance
d. Boswellia serrata

99. Hasbe zail me kaun se dawa Corrosive hai:
a. Zingaar
b. Baloot
c. Gile Miltani
d. Arosa

100. Jarahat Chashm me amale takhdeer ka istemaal sab se pahle kis Tabeeb ne kiya?
a. Abul Qasim Zohravi
b. Ibne zohar
c. Ibne Rushd
d. Ali bin Eesaa Kamal

101. The primary factor in resuscitation of a cardiac arrest patient is:
a. Cardiac compression
b. I.V Fluids
c. Adequate airway
d. Digitalis

102. Bilateral epitrocheal lymphadenopathy is seen in all except?
a. Syphilis
b. Tularemia
c. Toxoplasmosis
d. Sarcoidosis

103. Harners syndrome associated with pain in shoulder & arm is suggestive of:
a. Aortic aneurism

b. MI

c. Cervical spondilosis

d. Pancots tumor

104. The most common cause for recurrent laryngeal nerve palsy is:

a. Carotid body tumor

b. Thyroidectomy

c. Secondaries in neck

d. All of the above

105. Transpyloric passes through:

a. T12-L1

b. L5-S1

c. T10

d. L1-L2

106. Mandarja zail me se kaun sab se ziyadah good suture material hai:

a. Silk

b. Catgut

c. Cotton thread

d. Vicryl

107. Obstetricians hand kis marz me hota hai?

a. Hypothyroidism

b. Hypoparathyroidism

c. Hyperparathyroidism

d. None of the above

108. What is the colour of oxygen cylinder?

a. White

b. Grey

c. Blue

d. Black

109.Kochers method mandarja zail se mutaliq hai:

a. Cholecystectomy

b. Hipjoint reduction

c. Shoulder joint reduction

d. Elbow joint reduction

110. Carolis disease me biliary tree ka dilatation:

a. Congenital hota hai

b. Acquired hota hai

c. Traumatic hota hai

d. None of the above

111. Gallows splint kis umr me istemaal hota hai?

a. Infants

b. Paediatric

c. Geriatric

d. Adult

112. Proximal ulna ke fracture aur redial head ke dislocation ko kiya kahte hain?

a. Galezzia fracture

b. Montaggia fracture

c. Colles fracture

d. None of the above

113. Inta abdominal aur Extra abdominal swelling me kis test se faraq karte hain?

a. Carnetts test

b. Chair test

c. Parks test

d. None of the above

114. Undescended tests and retractile tests me kis sign se faraq karte hain?

a. Table test

b. Bed test

c. Chair test

d. All of the above

115. Small congenital hydrocoel ka ilaj kiya ho sakta hai?

a. Kisi ilaj ki zaroora nahi hai

b. Aspiration karna chhahiye

c. Corticisteroid injection se sookh jata hai

d. Operation

116. Ochner Sherrens regimen kis ke kiye sab se maozo ilaj hai hai?

a. Acute appendicitis

b. Appendicular abscess

c. Appendicular Mass

d. Chronic appendicitis

117. Courvoisier law is related to:

a. Jaundice

b. Carcinoma head of pancreas

c. Common bile duct stone

d. Allof the above

118. Fourniers gangrene occurs in:

a. Toes

b. Scrotum

c. Fingers

d. Muscles

119. Mallory weis tear occurs at:

a. Lower end of oesophagus

b. Gstro oesophageal junction

c. Upper oesophagus

d. Mid oesophagus

120. Regarding spermatocoel all is correct except?
a. Occurs in head of epidydimis
b. Contain barley water fluid
c. Tender
d. Contain spermatozoa

121. Serum amylase level is raised in all except?
a. Duodenal ulcer perforation
b. Pancreatitis
c. Appendicitis
d. Small bowel strangulation

122. Cullens sugn is seen in:
a. Acute cholecystitis
b. Acute gastritis
c. Acute hemorrhagic pancreatitis
d. Rupture of appendix

123. The best skin graft for open wound is:
a. Isograft
b. Homograft
c. Allograft
d. Autograft

124. Wound healing is worst in:
a. Sternum
b. Anterior neck
c. Eyelid
d. Lips

125. Laproscopic cholecystectomy ke liye peritoneal cavity me kaun se gas dali jati hai?
a. Oxygen
b. N oxide
c. Carbon monoxide
d. Carbon dioxide

126. Ketamine ka route of administration kiya hota hai?
a. I/M and I/V
b. I/V and Inhalation
c. I/M and Inhalation
d. Inhalation only

127. Hemorrhagic shock ka pahla clinical feature kiya hota hai?
a. Rised in blood pressure
b. Fall in blood pressure
c. Bradycardia
d. Tachycardia

128. Halothane anaesthesia se kiya pareshani ho sakti hai?
a. Rise in pulse rate and B.P both
b. Rise in pulse rate and fall inB.P
c. Rise in B.P and fall in pulse rate
d. Fall in pulse rate and B.P both

129. Epidural anaesthesia ke liye Bupivacaine kaha de jati hai?
a. Sub arachnoid spasce me
b. Ligamentum flavum
c. Extradural space
d. Spinal cord me

130. Spinal anaesthesia ke fauran bad in me kiya ho sakta hai?
a. Rise in B.P
b. Rise in H.R
c. Fall in B.P
d. None of the above

131. Neostigmine ka istemal kis liye hota hai?
a. Reversal of depolarizing muscle relaxant

b . Reversal of ether anaesthesia

c. Reversal of non depolarizing muscle relaxant

d. Reversal of intravenous anaesthesia

132. Kis muscle relaxant ke istemal se muscular fasciculation ho sakta hai?

a. Atracurium

b. Suxamethonium

c. Pancuronium

d. Tubocurarine

133. Junani zindagi me ghair navati kuryate hamara ke banana ka amal kis hafte se shuru ho jata hai?

a. 2nd weeks

b. 4th weeks

c. 8th weeks

d. 12th weeks

134. What is normal P-R interval?

a. 0.45 second

b. 0.35 second

c. 0.16 second

d . 0.11 second

135. Corticospinal Tract kis qism ka Tract hai?

a. Motor tract

b. Sensory tract

c. Both of them

d. None of them

136. Aldosterone ratoobat bainul khuliyat me izafa karta hai:

a. Ca++

b. K+

c. Cl-

d. Na+

137. Intrisic factor ka afraz kin khuliyat se hota hai:

a. Parietal cells se

b. Peptic cells se

c. Argentaffin cells se

d. Mucous cellsse

138. What is cause of Myasthenia Gravis?

a. Autoimmunity

b. Bacteria

c. Virus

d. None of the above

139. Alveoli me PO$_2$ kitna hota hai?

a. 100 mm of Hg

b. 104 mm of Hg

c. 95 mm of Hg

d. 40 mm of Hg

140. Azlate qlbia tetanized nahi hote hai is liye ki:

a. Is me pacemaker hota hai

b. In ka refractory period ziyadah hota hai

c. Yeh azlat shakht dar hote hai

d. In me slow Ca^{++}to Na+ channel hote hain

141. Kisi shakhs ka Hematocrit. 45% hai is ka matlab ye ha ki:

a. Plasma me 45% hamratuddam hai

b. Total khoon ka 45% plasma hai

c. Kurriyate hamarah me 45% hamratuddam hai

d. otal blood ka 45% kurriyate damawia hai

142. Action potential:

a. Ki intiha Na+ ke influx se hoti hai

b. Ki intiha K+ ke Efflux se hoti hai

c. Ki ibtida Na+ ke influx se hoti hai

d. Ki ibtida K+ ke influx se hoti hai

143. Concering the celiac trunk all the following statements are true except?
a. It supplies derivatives of fore gut
b. It arises from abdominal aorta at the level of disc between 1st lumber and 12th thoracic vertebrae
c. Itsspleenic branch supplies the duodenum
d. Its branches contribute to marginal artery

144. The structures passing through oesophageal opening of diaphragm are:
a. Oesophagus, Left gastric artery & phrenic artery
b. Oesophagus, Left gastric artery & Vagus nerve
c. Oesophagus, Vagus nerve & thoracic duct
d. None of the above

145. The redial nerve is directly related to:
a. Medial epicondyle of humerus
b. Spinal groove in shaft of humerus
c. Lateral epicondyle
d. Neck of humerus

146. All extrinsic and intrinsic muscles of the tongue are supplied by hypoglossus nerve except?
a. Hyoglossus
b. Platoglossus
c. Styloglossus
d. Genioglossus

147. The axillary nerve supplies:
a. Teres major and teres minor
b. Deltoid and teres minor
c. T and anconeus
d. Deltoid and levator scapulae

148. The superior epigastric artery is a branch of:
a. Internal thoracic artery
b. Subclavian artery
c. External iliac artery
d. Descending thoracic aorta

149. The mrdian nerve supplies the following muscle:
a. Flexor carpi ulnaris
b. Brachialis
c. Branchiradialis
d. Flexor digitorum sublimis

150. Winging of scapula is due to paralysis of:
a. Levator scapulae
b. Deltoid
c. Serratus anterior
d. Subscapularis

151. Small saphenous vein drains in to:
a. Great saphenous vein
b. Femoral vein in saphenous opening
c. Politeal vein
d. None of the above

152. The left testicular vein drains in to:
a. The left external iliac vein
b. IVC
c. The left interna iliac vein
D. Left renal vein

153. Bunyaadi dalak ki aqsam me darje zail nahi hai:
a. Dalak istedad
b. Dalak sulb
c. Dalak layyan
d. Dalak taveel

154. Mosam rabee ke shuru hone par zail tadbeer nihyat zaroori mazon hai:

a. Fasad aur Mushil ka intizaam

b. Riyazat aur ghiza me takhfeef

c. Hammam har ka istemal

d. Riyazat aur ghiza ki kasrat

155. Tadabeere mashaikh me kaun se darje zail tadbeer nahi shamil hai:

a. Martoob aur musakhin aghzia ka istemal

b. Dalak aur riyazat ka istemal

c. Mudriyaat ka istemal

d. Barid aghzia ka isteemal

156. Tadabeere itifal me 6 years ki umr ke children me darje zail tdbeer se mazon hai:

a. Hammam me takhfeef aur riyazat me kasrat

b. Hammam me kasrat aur riyazat me takhfee

c. Dono me takhfee

d. Dono me kasrat

157. Khoon ke mizaj ke liye munasib kaun sa mosam hai?

a.Khareef

b. Shitaa

c. Rabee

d. Saif

158. Hawae muheet rooh ke tabai mizaj ke muqable:

a. Bahut barid hoti hai

b. Bahut har hoti hai

c. Yaksa mizaj ki hoti hai

d. None of the above

159. Miqdaare warzish ke taaiyun ka taluque darje zail se nahi hai:
a. Jild kinrangat
b. Sans ki harkat
c. Paseena ki halat
d. Harkatte aza

160. Aghraze dalak me darje zail shamil nahi hai:
a. Naram azlaat ko sakht karna
b. Mote azlaat ko dubla karna
c. Aasab ko taqwwiat dena
d. Fuzlat dafa karne ke liye

161. Hammam karne ki kis halat me sudde ban ne ke imkaan hai:
a. Empty stomach
b. Full stomach
c. Both of the above
d. None of the above

162. Istifragh ghai tabai me darje zail halat nahi milti hai:
a. Quwwate dafia ka kamzoor ho jana
b. Quwwate masika ka kamzoor ho jana
c. Majari ka kushada ho jana
d. Quwwate hazima ka zaeef ho jana

163. What is chemical name of Vitamin B2?
a. Niacine
b. Pyridoxine
c. Riboflavin
d. Thiamine

164. Darje zail teeka marz se pahle nahi diya jata hai:
a. Measles vaccine
b. Typhoid vaccine
c. Rabies vaccine

d. None of the above

165. Which disease is not caused by Mosquitos?
a. Trichuriasis
b. Filiariasis
c. Japanese encephalitis
d. Yellow fever

166. Peshawarana longo ke liye radiation ki permissible limit darje zail hai:
a. 5 rems salana
b. 5 rems mahana
c. 10 rems salana
d. 10 rems mahana

167. Slow sand filter ka rate of filtration kitna hota hai:
a. 1-0.8 cu. Meter/sq.m
b. 0.4-4 cu. Meter/sq.m
c. 0.1-0.4 cu. Meter/sq.m
d. 0.2-0.8 cu. Meter/sq.m

168. What is daily requirement of iron in adult?
a. 0.9 mg
b. 0.3-0.9 mg
c. 0.9-15mg
d. 0.15-0.21 mg

169. Dengue fever is transmitted by:
a. Anopheles
b. Culex
c. Aedes
d. Mansonia

170. WHO ke kitne ilaaqai markaz hain?
a. 4
b. 5

c. 6
d. 7

171. P.H.C me new scheme ke mutabiq kitna staff hota hai?
a. 3 Member
b. 14 or 15 Member
c. 17 or 18 Member
d. 18 or 19 Member

172. ORS me darje zail shamil nahi hai:
a. Sodium chloride
b. Sodium citrate
c. Potassium chloride
d. Potassium citrate

173. What is incubation period of Tuberculosis?
a. 2-4 Weeks
b. 4-12 Weeks
c. 12-16 Weeks
d. 4-12 Months

174. Which of the following harmful things not present in water?
a. Flourine
b. Nitrate
c. PAH
D. Hydrogen sulphide

175. Paani ki safai me rolling boil ke liye waqt darker hota hai:
a. 1-5 minute
b. 1-5 hours
c. 5-10 second
d. 5-10 minute

176. WHO kis san me qaim hoa?
a. 1946
b. 1948
c. 1950
d. 1984

177. Gumma ki khusoosiyat hai ki ye zakhm:
a. Painful, shallow punchedout hota hai
b. Painful, deep undetermined edged hota hai
c. Painless, shallow undetermined hota hai
d .Painful, deep punchedout hota hai

178. Meighs syndrome me:
a. Fibroma of ovary, Hydrothorax and ascites hota hai
b. Uterine polyp, Hydrothorax and ascites hota hai
c. Uterine fibroid and ascites hota hai
d. Benign ovarian cyst and ascites hota hai

179. What is main cause of DUB?
a. Ovarian tumors
b. Uterine tumors
c. Anovulation
d. None of the above

180. Fothergills operation ke zarye kis ko durust kiya jata hai?
a. Cystocoele
b. Uterine prolapsed with cystocoele and Rectocoele
c. Rectocoele
d. Cystourethrocoele

181. Usre tams aur rataq kis qism ke reham me paye jate hain?
a. Uterus septus
b. Uterus unicornis
c. Bicornuate uterus

d. Hypoplastic uterus

182. What are broad ligaments?
a. True Ligaments
b. Peritoneal folda
c. Muscular bands
d. Fibrous bands

183. Bacterial vaginosis ka causative organism kaun sa hai?
a. Candida albiicans
b. Gardenella vaginalis
b. Gardenella vaginosis
d. Trepenoma palladium

184. Which is most common pelvic tumor found in female?
a. Leiomyoma
b. Choriocarcinoma
c. Chindroma
d. Blastoma

185. Extra uterine presence of endometrial glands and stroma ko kahte hai:
a. Endometritis
b. Endometriosis
c. Endometrial hyperplasia
d. None of them

186. What is Osteoporosis?
a. Decreased bone mass
b. Holes in bones
c. Both of the above
d. None of the above

187. During pregnancy which malignancy is most common?
a. Carcinoma of vagina
b. Carcinoma of uterus
c. Breast cancer
d. Cervical cancer

188. HELLP Syndrome kis disease ka complication hai?
a. Chronic nephritis
b. Severe pre eclampsia
c. Hypovolumic shock
d. Anemia

189. X-ray me confirmed death ke kiya sign hai?
a. Overlapping of cranial bone
b. Hyperflextion of vertebral column
c. Gas bubble in the heart
d. All of the above

190. Neural tube defect is caused due to deficiency of:
a. Vitamin A deficiency
b. Vitamin D deficiency
c. Iron deficiency
d. Folic acid deficiency

191. Extra embryonic mesoderm ko kiya kahte hai:
a. Primary mesoderm
b. Secondary mesoderm
c. Tertiary mesoderm
d. None of the above

192. Fetal development ke kis din amniotic cavity banti hai?
a. 15th day
b. 10th day

c. 5th day
d. 8th day

193. Janeen ko embryo hamal ki kis muddat me kahte hain?
a. 3rd month-4th month
b. 15th day-9th week
c. 8th week-10th week
d. None of them

194. Pelvic cavity ka anterio-posterio diameter kiya hota hai?
a. 11 cm
b. 10 cm
c. 12 cm
d. 13 cm

195. Fetus compressus ko aur kiya kahte hai?
a. Fetus papyraceous
b. Super fetation
c. Compression syndrome
d. None of the above

196. Pregnancy ke dauran blood volume kitne percent barh jata hai?
a. 30-50%
b. 20%
c. 15%
d. 25%

197. Complete breech ko kahte hai:
a. Frank breech
b. Flexed breech
c. Breech with extended legs
d. None

198. Defective Mullerian fusion ki wajah se kiya kharabi paidahoti hai?
a. Double uterus
b. Septate uterus
c. Both
d. None

199. Interstitial implantation poori tarah hota hai:
a. 16th day
b. 11th day
c. 20th day
d. 28th day

200. Ovum ke chharo taraf hota hai:
a. Vitelline membrane
b. Perivitelline membrane
c. Both
d. None

MD AMU ENTRANCE EXAMNATION
ANSWER KEY 2009-10

1. B   2. A   3. D   4. D   5. D
6. B   7. A   8. C   9. A   10. A
11. C   12. D   13. A   14. D   15. D
16. A   17. B   18. A   19. A   20. C
21. D   22. B   23. C   24. A   25. D
26. A   27. D   28. A   29. D   30. B
31. B   32. C   33. A   34. B   35. D
36. C   37. D   38. A   39. C   40. D
41. A   42. A   43. C   44. B   45. A
46. A   47. A   48. D   49. B   50. C
51. C   52. C   53. C   54. A   55. D
56. D   57. C   58. B   59. A   60. C
61. B   62. D   63. B   64. A   65. A
66. D   67. B   68. A   69. B   70. D
71. D   72. D   73. B   74. B   75. C
76. C   77. A   78. D   79. C   80. A
81. D   82. C   83. A   84. D   85. C
86. B   87. C   88. A   89. A   90. C
91. C   92. B   93. A   94. D   95. C
96. A   97. A   98. A   99. A   100.A
101.C   102.A   103.C   104.D   105.A
106.D   107.B   108.D   109.C   110.A
111.B   112.B   113.A   114.C   115.D
116.C   117.A   118.B   119.B   120.C
121.C   122.C   123.D   124.A   125.D
126.A   127.D   128.D   129.A   130.C
131.C   132.B   133.B   134.C   135.A
136.D   137.A   138.A   139.A   140.B
141.D   142.B   143.D   144.B   145.B
146.B   147.D   148.A   149.D   150.C
151.C   152.D   153.A   154.A   155.D
156.C   157.C   158.A   159.B   160.D
161.B   162.D   163.C   164.C   165.A

166.A 167.C 168.A 169.C 170.C
171.B 172.D 173.A 174.D 175.D
176.B 177.D 178.A 179.A 180.B
181.C 182.B 183.B 184.A 185.B
186.C 187.D 188.B 189.D 190.D
191.A 192.D 193.B 194.C 195.A
196.A 197.B 198.C 199.B 200.A

1. Fikr yaani sooch kitni quwwa se Murakkab hai?
a. 2
b. 3
c. 4
d. 5

2. Baraz me ratubat zyada hona dalalat karta hai?
a.Kasrat Akhlat
b.Kasrat Reeh
c.Kasrat Ratubat
d.Sue Hazam

3. Ajzae boul ki nauyiat kiya hai?
a. Mayi wa aarzi
b. Mayi wa zardi
c. Mayi wa arzi
d. Mayi wa juzwi

4. Takhalkhul means:
a.Hawa ka dakhil hona
b.Miqdar me badhne ko
c.Hajam me badhne ko
d. A, B & C

5. Ghiza ko hazam karne ke liye kiya lazim hai?
a. Istifraghe mawad
b. Ehtabas mawad
c. Tanqia mawad
d. Tasfia mawad

6. Sukoon ki ziyadti badan me kiya paida karti hai?

a. Hararat

b. Baroodat

c. Ratoobat

d. Yaboosat

7. Asbabe sitta zarooryia fourth sabab kaun hai?

a. Ehtabas wa istifragh

b. Naum wa yaqza

c. Harkat wa sukoone badani

d. Harkat wa sukoone nafsani

8. Halate Salisa ka nazarya kis Hakeem ka hai?

a. Buqrat

b. Jalinoos

c. Ibne Zakaria

d. Ibne Sina

9. Afal Adwia is determined by:

a. Wo afal jo bahalat marz hote hain

b. Wo afal jo bahalat sehat hote hain

c. Wo afal jo la marz wa la sehat hote hain

d. A, B & C

10. Kin amraz me nuzaj ki qataan zaroorat nahi hai:

a. Amraze damwia

b. Amraze Balghamia

c. Amraze Safrawia

d. Amraze Saudawia

11. Darajat ul Adwia is determined with:

a. Miqdar khurak

b. Miqdar tasir

c. Mizaj

d. A, B & C

12. Ilme Tibb ki bunyaad kis nazariya par hai?

a. Aag, paani, hawa, mitti par hai

b. Anasire arba par hai

c. Teen anasir oar hai

d. Anasire kasira par hai

13. Fasad ek kulli istifragh ha kyon ki:

a. Ye kul amraz me mustamil hai

b. Ye kul akhlat ka istifragh karta hai

c. Ye kul zarai istifragh par muheet hai

d. Ye kul mawad ko jism se kharij karta hai

14. Balgham ke istifragh ke liye kaun sa zariya bahtar hai:

a. Qai

b. Fasad

c. Hajamat

d. Ishal

15. Ghizai kaseef qalilul taghzia raddiul kemoos:

a. Batakh ka gost

b. Saag

c. Lungs

d. Sookha gost

16. Hifz sehat ke liye mahine me do bar qai karna chhiye kis ka nazariya hai?

a. Razi

b. Saikh

c. Jalinoos

d. Buqrat

17. Zakhira khuwarzam Shahi ka musanif:

a. Mohammad Husain Sherazi

b. Abul Qasim Farishta

c. Ismail Jirjani

d. Sadeeduldeen garvi

18. Tabiyate insaan ka musanif kaun hai?

a. Razi

b. Ibne Butlan

c. Buqrat

d. Aladkhuwar

19. Fadagh kahte hai:

a. Shiryan ke tafaruqe ittesal ko

b. Azlat ke tafaruqe ittesal ko

c. Aasab ke tafaruqe ittesal ko

d. Aghshia ke tafaruqe ittesal ko

20. Mooti jharrah ka madda kis qism ka hota hai?

a. Balghami

b. Safrawi

c. Damwi

d. Balghame affan wa Safra ka amizah

21. Kis marz ke jaresheem ko acid fast stain se rangte hai?

a. Juzam

b. Diq

c. Sartan

d. Sarsam

22. Boul Ashab qism hai:

a. Boule sabz ki

b. Boule surkh ki

c. Boule zarad ki

d. Boule siyah ki

23. Aqsarai ka musanif kaun hai?

a. Ali Husain Ghilani

b. Mohammad Amli

c. Jamaluddin

d. Alauddin

24. Unsure khizreen kis qism se taluq rakhta hai hai?

a. Ubsure hawai se

b. Ubsure naar se

c. Ubsure maai se

d. Ubsure arzi se

25. Baiza kis ke liye mustamil hai?

a. Khoon

b. Balgham

c. Safra

d. Sauda

26. Manai Ufoonat kaun si khilt hoti hai?

a. Khilte dam

b. Khilte safra

c. Khilte balgham

d. Khilte sauda

27. Quwwai mudarka taadad me kitne hote hain?

a. 2

b. 5

c. 3

d. 10

28. Desqooredos ne kaun se kitab tasneef ki hai?

a. Kitabul Akhlat

b. Kitabul Haahaish

c. Kitabul Nabzul kabir

d. Kitabul Kiuliyat

29. Hakeem Ajmal khan ka inteqaal kaha hoa?

a. Delhi

b. Frans

c. Rampur

d. New delhi

30. Ghazroof Mukbi ke fail ko kis ne wazah kiya?

a. Jalinoos

b. Herophilus

c. Ersataratos

d. Ibne Hubal Baghdadi

31. Hindi Tibb me tashkhees ke kitne zarai hai?

a. 3

b. 5

c. 8

d. 10

32. Alqanoon fit tib ki all five volumes ka urdoo tarzuma kis ne kiya?

a. Khuwaza Rizwan

b. Allama Kabiruddin

c. Allama Ghulam Husain Kantoori

d. Hakeem Hadi Husain

33. Damshaq me Juzamio ke liye makhsoos shifa khana kis ne qaim kiya ?

a. Khalifa ameer Maavia

b. Khalifa Mansoor

c. Khalifa valeed bin Abdul Malik

d. Khalifa Mamoon Rasheed

34. Hazal zohari ka amooman sabab hai:

a. Suzak

b. Aatishk

c. Wajau zohar

d. Zoaf aasab

35. Naqras ki ibtida kis azu me pahle waqai hoti hai?

a. Haath ki ungiliyo ke joro me

b. Khutne ke jor me

c. Paeer ke ungothe me

d. Pusht ke moharo ke jor me

36. Sudee barid sazij ke ilaj ke liye:

a. Sandal safed aur kafoor ka lap kare

b. Roghane gul aur sirka kapre me tar karke sar par rakhe

c. Arqe khas arqe kewra mila kar lakhlakha soonghai

d. Garam kapre urha kar garam paani ka bhapara de

37. Metastasis kis enzyme se asani se hoti hai?

a. Metalloprotinase

b. Phopholipase

c. Pepsin

d. Prostglandin

38. Huroor kis marz ka naam hai?

a. Humme Matbaqa

b. Loo laghna

c. Nazla haar

d. None of the above

39. Shiryaan ka character and volume sab se bahtar kha dekha ja sakta hai

a. Carotid artery:

b. Branchial artery

c. Femoral artery

d. Radial artery

40. Arteriosclerosis me khoon me kis ki miqdaar barh jati hai?

a. Protein

b. RBCs

c. Cholestrol

d. Vitamin B12

41. What are the causes of Spleenomeghaly?
a. Malaria
b. Epstein Barr Viral Infection
c. Acute nephritis
d. Only a and b

42. Best specimen of bone for sex determination is:
a. Femur
b. Pelvis
c. Skull
d. Mandible

43. Small pulse volume kis me hota hai?
a. Cardiac failure
b. Essential hypertension
c. PDA
d. All of the above

44. Marawwaqain khas dawa hai:
a. Warme kabid ki
b. Suddae kabid ki
c. Mooti jhharra ki
d. Sarsam ki

45. Normal PR interval:
A. 0.8 to 1second
b. 0.12 to 0.2 second
c. 0.11 to 0.12 second
d. None of the above

46. Ye marz naujawan girls me haiz ki kharabi ki wajah se hota hai:
a. Piles
b. Khizra
c. Natourreham
d. Seelannurreham

47. Clubbing of finger me kiya hota hai?
a. Nails become brittle
b. Nails become concave
c. Nails loose, longitudinal ridges
d. None of the above

48. Natroonab kis ko kahte hai?
a. Maul zubn ko
b. Gulab ko
c. Ma usshaeer ko
d. Soda paani ko

49. Advia ki wajah se hone wali nausea and vomiting me kaun centre stimulate hota hai?
a. Dopamine receptor
b. Histamine e receptor
c. Cholinergic receptor
d. Both a and c

50. Nazla muzmin ki khas dawa hai:
a. Khamira gaiozaban ambari wa itrifal ustukhuddos
b. Khamira murvareed wa itrifal saghir
c. Khamira sandal wa itrifal kabir

d. Khamira abresham sada wa itrifal mundi

51. Main cause of arteriosclerosis is:
a. Alcohol
b. Cigrett
c. Starvation
d. Bisyarkhori

52. Crohns disease ka asal sabab hai:
a. Bacterial infection
b. Ghizai beatidali
c. Zahni dabao
d. None of the above

53. Prolonged bed rest ka aam complication hai:
a. Arterial embolism
b. Cerebral embolism
c. Deep vein thrombosis
d. All of the above

54. Warme gurda haad me paya jata hai:
a. Humme lazima
b. Humme mukhtalta
c. Humme naiba
d. Humme Yaum

55. Budahape ki halat me zaufe bah ke liye muzarrab hai:
a. Majoon Nankhawah
b Majoon Mocharas
c. Majoon Aarad khurma

d. Laboobe kabir

56. Fallots tetralogy me kiya paya jata hai?
a. Pulmonary stenosis
b. VSD
c. ASD
d. Both a and b

57. Lasarghas kahte hai:
a. Sarsame Safrawi ko
b. Sarsame Balghami ko
c. Sarsame Saudawi ko
d. Sarsame Damwi ko

58. Klinefelters syndrome ka karyotype kiya hai:
a. 47 XXY
b. 46 XY
c. XXY
d. XYY

59. Achanak naaf ke itiraff shaded dard hota hai baraz aur riyah ka akhraj nahi ho pata qai aati hai kis marz me:
a. Qoolanj kulve me
b. Sudda aama me
c. Qoolanj kabdi me
d. Gastric ulcer me

60. Syndrome X kis me hota hai?
a. D.M
b. Renal failure
c. M.I

d. Testicular atrophy

61. The first tooth to appear is:
a. First molar
b. Lateral incisor
c. Upper canine
d. Lower central incisor

62. ECG ki Lead I me kis ke beech me connection hota hai?
a. Right arm- Right leg
b. Right arm- Left leg
c. Right arm- left arm
d. Left arm- left leg

63. Type I diabetes kis virus se ho sakta hai?
a. Coxsakie B4
b. Coxsakie B2
c. Hepto virus
d. None of the above

64.Cell membrane kis madda ki bani hoti hai?
a. Lecithin
b. Phospholipid
c. Mucophospolipid
d. None of rhe above

65. Garam dawao ke istemaal se kis qism ka dard e sar aariz hota hai?
a. Sudaee Damwi
b. Sudaee Safarawi
c. Sudaee Har sazaj

d. Sudaee Shirki

66. Marz Asaaba kaseerul waqoo hai:
a. Childrens me
b. Womens me
c. Adhar umr walon me
d. Old age me

67. Rewanchini ek mishal hai:
a. Mufaradul quwwa dawa ki
b. Murakkabul quwwa dawa ki
c. Quwwal amal dawa ki
d. Taseere Oola rakhne wali dawa

68. Parental route (Intravenous) se dawa jism me dakhil karne par lahique ho sakta hai:
a. Embolism
b. Thrombosis
c. Abscess
d. Paralysis

69. Jild par faili taseer rakhne wali ek aesi dawa jo muariqe arq amal karti hai:
a. Rasoot
b. Tukhm Khashkhash
c. Ajwain khurasaani
d. Afyun

70. Ek C.N.S Stimulant dawa ki mishal hai:
a. Ajwain
b. Beikh Luffah

c. Afyun

d. Izaraqi

71. Calcium jis dawa me Iron ke saath milkar paya jata hai:

a. Shangaraf

b. Murwareed

c. Sadaf sadiq

d. Busta ahmar

72. Dawa jo khoon se sauda ki ghair tabai ghilzat ko door karti hai:

a. Tukhm khurfa

b. Aftimoon

c. Tukhm Kaho

d. Sadaf sokhta

73. Ek mazeed laban dawa hai:

a. Habbul Qillt

b.Baboona

c. Khusk dana

d. Panbadana

74. Amber coloured watery discharge is sign of:

a. Ca. Fallopian Tube

b. Salpingitis

c. Parametritis

d. Para ovarin cyst

75. Mako ka mutradif name kiya hai?

a. Bazarulbanj

b. Bazarulkham

c. Khusyatul Salab

d. Inabul salab

76. Dawaul Misk is a type of:

a. Majoon

b. Khamira

c. Mufarrah

d. All

77. Zanjabeel me tez mazah (pungent taste) hota hai:

a. Ginger oil ki waja se

b. Gingerin ki waja se

c. Mucilage ki waja se

d. Starch ki waja se

78. Johare kemivia Starcinine ka sab se ziyadah muzir asar hota hai:

a. Spinal nerve par

b. Peripheral nerve par

c. Nerve fibre par

d. Cardiac muscle par

79. Qatai aadate afyun nihayet Mujarrab murakkab Hai:

a. Majoon Najah

b. Majoon Izaraqi

c. Jawarish jalinoos

d. Habbe jadwar

80.Chhar tukhm me shamil tukhm ke naam:

a. Tukhm kanocha, tukhm kata, tukhm khiyarza, tukhm kaddu

b. Tukhm bartang, tukhm rehaan tukhm gazar, tukhm aspaghol

c. Tukhm kanocha, tukhm kharpaza tukhm bartang, tukhm sibat

d. Tukhm kanocha, tukhm aspaghol tukhm bartang, tukhm rehaan

81. Tareeq Lolabi is:
a. Bhodar jantar
b. Damru jantar
c. Nadi jantar
d. Doli jantatr

82. Kameela kiya hai:
a. Flower
b. Fruit
c. Barg
d. None of the above

83.Beesh ki Miqdare khurak batai:
a. 250mg- 500mg
b. 100mg- 200mg
c. 50mg- 100mg
d. 25mg- 50mg

84. Kis dawa ko muddabar karne ke liye Ghirbaal istemaal hoti hai?
a. Qaranulain
b. Kholanjan

c. Ghariqoon

d. Mazriyoon

85. Kitabul Havi alkabir ke kis jild me dawao ka zikr haii?

a. 4th and 5th volume

b. 10th and 11th volume

c. 17th and 18th volume

d. 21th and 22th volume

86. Zeeqanafs me mufeed murakkab hai:

a. Sharbate Dinar

b. Sharbate Zofa

c. Sharbate Unnab

d. Sharbate Neelofar

87. Salilic acid paya jata hai:

a. Nakhoona me

b. Baboona me

c. Asgandh me

d. Bozidaan me

88. Saalab mishri ka kaun sa hissa istemaal hota hai:

a. Tukhm

b. Gums

c. Branch

d. Root

89. Which is antioxidant?

a. Rewandchini

b. Kharkhusk

c. Suddab

d. Saatar

90. Kis tarah ki dawai prostaglandin ki synthesis ko rokti hai:

a. NSAID

b. Suphonamides

c. Antibiotics

d. Antihistamine

91. Oodsaleeb kiya hai?

a. Fruit

b. Flower

c. Root

d. Stem

92. Kushta Qalai ki shanakth kya hai?

a. Aag me dalne se dhuwan nahi deta

b. Aag me dalne se dhuwan nahi deta

c. Barg mudar me peesne se chamak deti

d. Aab sada par teerta hai

93. Zeera safed kis family se taluque hai?

a. Labiatae

b. Polygonaceae

c. Papilionacae

d. Umbelliferae

94. Kalaunji ka kaunsa juz batoore dawa istemal hota hai:

a. Fruit

217

b. Flower

c. Tukhm

d. Shagofa

95. Darchikna murakkab hai:

a. Nausader aur gile Armani ka

b. Shibbe yamaani aur semab ka

c. Kibreet, gile Armani aur sammaulfar ka

d. Simaab aur sammulfaar ka

96. Hadtal belongs to:

a. Anfas

b. Ahjar

c. Arwah

d. Falzat

97. Bora Armani ka badal hai:

a. Bozidaan

b. Hilteet

c. Turmus

d. Suhaga

98. Dawa Jharh ka tareeqa istemaal:

a. Humool

b. Zimad

c. Tial

d. Latookh

99. Qawaneen Advia se mutaalique kitab ka name hai:

a. Kitabul Shamil

b. Kitabul Hashaish

c. Kitabul Tasreef

d. Kitabul Havi alkabir

100. Naak ke ghar ka dangerous area kahlata hai:

a. Littles area

b. Olfactory area

c. Vestibular area

d. Turbinal area

101. Seltingsun sign kis condition ki alamat hai:

a. Hydrocephalus

b. Thyrotoxicosis

c. Terminal stage of malignancy

d. Neurogenic shock

102. Heart me increase filling pressure kis condition me hota hai:

a. Hypovolumic shock

b. Cardiogenic shock

c. Septic shock

d. Neurogenic shock

103. Bleeding apne aap kaha se nahi rukti hai:

a. Capillaries

b. Larger vein

c. Medium sized arteies

d. Medium sized veins

104. Jarahat chashm me amal takhdeer ka istemaal sab se pahle kis Tabeeb ne kiya:

a. Ibne Zohar

b. Ibne Rushd

c. Abul Qasim Zohravi

d. Ali bin Easaa Kamal

105. Eye me corneal reflex kab ghaib hota hai?

a. Inferior orbital nerve ke jarahat ki soorat me

b. Ophthalmic nerve ke jarahat ki soorat me

c. Trigeminal motor nerve ke jarahat ki soorat me

d. Cilliary ganglion ke jarahat ki soorat me

106. Ulcer ki everted edges kis tarah ke ulcer me milti hai:

a. Malignant ulcer

b. Rodent t ulcer

c. Tuberculous ulcer

d. Trophic ulcer

107. Implantation dermoid kaha par hota hai?

a. Palm

b. Finger

c. Sole

d. All of the above

108. Kis umr me water excess ki waja se convulsion ho jate hai?

a. Infants

b. Children

c. Middle age

d. Elderly

109. Bar bar stomach me dard, jaundice and fever kis marz ki alamat hai?

a. Stone in CBD

b. Hepatitis

c. Cancer pancreas

d. Cholangio carcinoma

110. Stomach ke kis hisse me cancer common hai?

a. Fundus

b. Body

c. Antrum

d. None of the above

111. Papillitis kis jagah ki bimari hai?

a. Optic nerve head

b. Optic nerve

c. Optic radiation

d. All of the above

112. Spinal anaesthesia kis jagahdiya jata hai?

a. Spinal cord

b. Eztradural spaces

c. Intadural spaces

d. Ventral column

113. Peptic ulcer is common in which part of duodenum?

a. 1st

b. IInd

c. IIIrd

d. 4TH

114. Epiglottis me maut ka sabab hai:
a. Acute laryngitis
b. Septicaemia
c. Respiratory obstruction asphyxia
d. None of the above

115. Anaesthesia me ether ka istemal kis san me shuru hoa?
a. 1884
b. 1847
c. 1984
d.1857

116. Carbuncle jism ke kis hissa me ziyadah hota hai?
a. Palm
b. Sole
c. Back
d. Chest

117. Ragi is a richest source of:
a. Iron
b. Protein
c. Calcium
d. Cabohydrate

118. Hypopadius me urethra ki opening kaha nahi hoti hai?
a. Dorsum of penis
b. Ventral surface of corona

c. Ventral suface of body of penis

d. Ventral surface of colum

119. Septic shock ki waja:

a. Bacteria

b. Viruses

c. Fungi

d. All of the above

120. Acute appendicitis me maximum tenderness kis jaga hoti hai?

a. Umblicous

b. Mc Burneys point

c. Right hypochondrium

d. Supra pubic region

121. Hernia ke sab se serous complication kiya hai?

a. Increase in size

b. Irreducibility

c. Strangulation

d. Obstruction

122. Burn patients ke marne ki aham waja hai:

a. Hupovolumic shock

b. Chocking

c. Septicaemic shock

d. Rt heart failure

123. Which of the following is related to Rokitanski-Kuster Huauser Syndrome?

a. Cryptomenorrhoea

b. Amenorrhoea

c. Dysmenorrhoea

d. DUB

124. Dehydration me urine ki specific gravity par kiya asar padta hai?

a. Increased

b. decreased

c. Does not change

d. Remains normal

125. McIndole's and Williiam's surgery are the choice in:

a. Inqilab ur Raham

b. Bawasir Reham

c. Inshiqaq ur Reham

d. Rataq

126. Chocholate Cysts of the Ovary is a sign of:

a. Usr Tams Sanawi

b. Tahat Tams

c. Ta'ddud Tams

d. Kasrat Tams

127. Metrostaxis is a type of:

a. Metrorrhagia

b. Menorrhagia

c. Epimenorrhoea

d. Oligomenorrhoea

128. Ilaj bilyad ko kiya kahte hai?

a. Moalijat

b. Ilmul amraz

c. Ilmul jarahat

d. Ilmul Advia

129. Subcutaneous tissue aur muscle ko jorne ke liye aam taur par:

a. Catgut used

b. Silk used

c. Prolene used

d. Vicryl used

130. Small congenital hydrocele:

a. One year no treatment is needed

b. Operation is needed

c. Aspiration

d. Corticisteroid injection

131. Breast lump hone par fauran:

a. X-ray chest karana chhayie

b. C.T Scan karana chhayie

c. Mamography karana chhayie

d. F.N.A.C karana chhayie

132. Low back pain ke asbab hai:

a. Lumbo-sacral strain

b. Sacrol-illiac strai

c. Prolapsed intervertebral disc

d. None of the above

133. Dam me Co2 khaas taur par kis ke zariye transport hota hai:
a. Bicarbonate
b. Carbmino compound
c. Free Co2
d. Plasma protein combination

134. Gout ek disorder hai:
a. Purine metabolism
b. Pyrimidine metabolism
c. Oxalate metabolism
d. Protein metabolism

135. Pancreas ke delta cells se secrete hota hai:
a. Glucagon
b. Insulin
c. Somatostatin
d. Pancreatic polymerase

136. Ek baar sans lene me kitni Oxygen istemal hoti hai?
a. 300-400 c.c
b. 400-500 c.c
c. 200-300 c.c
d. 50-100 c.c

137. Ek din me Glomeruli se water filter hita hai:
a. 170 liters
b. 100 liters
c. 90 liters
d. 60 liters

138. Plasma aur serum me kiya faraq hai?

a. Lymphocyte

b. Clotting factor

c. RBC

d. All of the above

139. 24 hours me kitna urine banana zaroori hai excretion ke liye:

a. 100-200 ml

b. 400-500 ml

c. 1000 ml

d. None of the above

140. Rozana ek 70 kg marad ko kitne paani ki zaroorat hoti hai:

a. 1 liters

b. 2.5 liters

c. 3 liters

d. 4 liters

141. Serum potassium ka normal level kiya hota hai?

a. 1-3 mml/L

b. 3.5-5 mml/L

c. 5-7 mml/L

d. 7-10 mml/L

142. Nabz Zanabul Far me Ikhtilaf hota hai:

a. Azam wa Sighar

b. Quwwat wa Zayeef

c. Surat wa Batu

d. All

143. Nabz Tabai is seen as:

a. Azeem, Qawi and Mastawi

b. Mastawi, Munazzam and Saree

c. Mastawi, Munazzam and Jaiadul wazan

d. Mastawi, Munazzam, Jaiadul wazan and Qawi

144. Sebaceous cyst aam tur par jism ke kis hissa me paya jata hai?

a. Scalp

b. Neck

c. Chest

d. Abdomen

145. Left gastric artey kis ki branch hai:

a. Aorta

b. Coeliac artrey

c. Superir mesenteric artery

d. Inferior mesenteric artery

146. Sciatic nerve ka shumaar:

a. Big nerve me hota hai

b. Intermediate nerve me hota hai

c. Small nerve me hota hai

d. Taweel wa daqeeq nerve me hota hai

147. Konsa sabab, Sabab Muqawwama hai:

a. Shidat zaroorat

b. Qiwam Aala

c. Qalb ki harkat

d. All of the above

148. Kadurat se murad:

a. Wo halat jis me roshni na guzar sake

b. Wo halat jis me roshni guzar sake

c. Wo halat jo dekhne se gadla lage

d. A, B & C

149. Apex of heart banti hai:

a. Left atrium and small part of right atrium

b. Left ventricle

c. Right and left ventricle

d. Only left atrium

150. Kis marz me siyah qarura bura hai?

a. Amraz Kabid

b. Amraz Tihal

c. Amraz Qalb

d. Amraz Kulya wa Masana

151. Ghee ki tarah sufaid qarurah ko kehte hain?

a. Mukhati

b. Dasmi

c. Ihali

d. Nuqai

152. Ek baligh dimagh ka average weight hota hai:

a. 1250gm

b. 1300gm

c. 1400gm

d. 1500gm

153. Vomiting centre is present in:

a. Hypothalamus

b. Cerebellum

c. Pons

d. Medulla

154. Marz muzmin me Gurdon me bol hota hai:

a. Jhag der tak rehta hai

b. Jhag jald tut jata hai

c. Jhag zyada na paida hote hain

d. Jhag kam paida hote hain

155. Ophthalmic Neonatorum ka sabab hai:

a. Suzaki jarshoma

b. Trichomonas

c. Satreptococci

d. Niacin

156.Vertical transmission kis ke zariye hota hai?

a. Mosquitise

b. Fleas

c. Placenta

d. Toota

157. Agar ek baccha ka paidaishi wazan 3 kg hai to aam taur se ek year me iska wazan avwrage kam se kam kitna hoga?

a. 6 kg

b. 9 kg

c. 12.kg

d.15 kg

158. At the time birth what is length of Hindustani children is?

a. 40 cm

b. 50 cm

c. 60 cm

d. 70 cm

159. Extra calorie requirement of lactating mother is:

a. 100-150

b. 400-550

c. 700-850

d.None of the above

160. Dengue fever is transmitted by:

a. Anopheles

b. Culex

c. Aedes

d. Monsonoids

161. Presumptive coliform test is done in:

a. Cholera

b. Typhoid fever

c. Plague

d. Water

162. Iron deficiency anaemia kis ko kahte hai:

a. Micrcytic anaemia

b. Macrcytic anaemia

c. Hypodermic anaemia

d. None of the above

163. Hindustan me Anapheles Mosquitose ki kul kitni species payi jati hai:

a. 60

b. 55

c. 50

d. 45

164. Kitabi al Hawia wal Miya wal buldaan kis ki tasneef hai:

a. Jalinoos

b. Seikh bu ali Sina

c. Buqrat

d. Zakaria Razi

165. Casala collar kis ki deficiency se hota hai?

a. Riboflavin

b. Niacin

c. Thiamine

d. None of the above

166. Family planning ke liye mustamil calendar methods sab se pahle kis ne banaya?

a. Ogino

b. Ogawa

c. Osaka

d. None of the above

167. Multiperous women me contraceptive ke liye sab se mahooz tareeqa:

a. Oral pills

b. IUCD

c. Safe period

d. All

168. Planning committee and health survey kis naam se jani jati hai?

a. Mudalia committee

b. Chadha committee

c. Mukherji committee

d. None of the above

169. Transmission of infection ki chain me shamil nahi hai:

a. Source or reservoir

b. Environment

c. Mode of transmission

d. Susceptible host

170. Incubation period of Polio:

a. 3- 7 days

b. 7-14 days

c. 14-21 days

d. None of the above

171. Which of the following is Muzir Dimagh?

a. Ispaghol

b. Haleela Kabuli

c. Gundana

d. Suranjan

172. Neonatal period is:

a. Ist 52 days

b. Ist 65 days

c. Ist 38 days

d. Ist 28 days

173. Class room ke liye bahtar desk hota hai:

a. Negative desk

b. Positive desk

c. Aarzi desk

d. Zeero desk

174. Water borne disease is:

a. Chiken pox

b. Tetanus

c. Bacillary dysentery

d. Tuberculosis

175. Wah kaun se Vitamin hai jis se jism me Ca and Phophate ka absorption increase ho jata hai?

a. Vit. B12

b. Vit. D

c. Vit. A

d. Vit. B

176. Ishal ke ziyadah tar cases ka sabab hota hai:

a. Bateria

b. Protozoans

c. Viruses

d. None of the above

177. Hamale kazib me tammam alamate payi jati hai except?

a. Shikam ka barh jana

b. Nausea and vomiting

c. Amenorrhoea

d. Enlagement of uterus

178. Tamasi daur ke average din hote hai:

a. 26 days

b. 27 days

c. 32 days

d. 28 days

179. Duration of sperm capacitation:

a. 2-4 hours

b. 1-2 hours

c. 6-8 hours

d. 24 hours

180. Nauzayadah me tashanuj ka aam sabab:

a. Chot lgna

b. Shakar ki kami

c. Naseem ki kami

d. Ca ki kami

181. Witches milk kiya hai:

a. Milk from baby's breast

b. Milk from mother's breast

c. All of the above

d. None of the above

182. Menopause ke baad Gonadotrophins kab tak badhe rahte hai?

a. Rest of life

b. 2 years

C. 1 year

d. 6 months

183. During lactation which drug is contraindicated?

a. Iron

b. Calcium

c. Metronidazole

d. None

184. Premature rupture of membrane kab kaha jata hai?

a. Before second stage of labour

b. Rupture onset of labour

c. After 36 weeks

d. None of the above

185. Daurane hamal nabz me hasbe zail tabdeli hoti hai:

a. Saree,mutwatir and azim

b. Azim

c. Batee aur mutwatir

d. Minshari

186. Neonatal death kise kahte hai?

a. 6 Weeks after birth

b. 10 Weeks after birth

c. 4 Weeks after birth

d. 2nd day after birth

187. Source of relaxin is:

a. Medulla

b. Pituitary gland

c. Placenta

d. Adrenal cortex

188. Jisme asfar ka asfar rang kis wajah se hota hai?

a. Cholestin

b. Carotene

c. Serum

d. Blood

189. During Puberty in which stage the breast development occurs?

a. Pre puberty Stage *

b. 1st stage of puberty

c. 2nd stage of puberty

d. 3rd stage of puberty

190. Following hormones are secreted from palcenta except?

a. Estrogen

b. Progetron

c. H.C.G

d. F.H.S

191. Copper T kis tarah act karti hai?

a. Inhibiting ovulation

b. Causin aseptic endometritis

c. Decreased cervical mucus

d. All of the above

192. Kopliks spot sab se pahle kaha jahir hota hai?

a. Inner cheek opposite 2nd molar

b. Opposite 3rd molar

c . opposite 1st molar

d. None of the above

193. What is prophylactic dose of folic acid?

a. 5 mg TDS

b. 5 mg OD

c. 5 mg QID

d. 5 mg BD

194. Fetal skull ka longest diameter kesa hota hai?

a. Occipito frontal

b. Mento vertical

c. Sub occipito bregmatic

d. Sub mento vertical

195. Asphyxia livida me apgar score kitna hota hai?

a. 4-6

b. 0-4

c. 4-5

d. 9-10

196. Hypothalamic amenorrhoea ki aam wajah:

a. Sheehan syndrome

b. Kallman syndrome

c. Asherman syndrome

d. None of the above

197. Choriocarcinoma ka marker kiya hai?

a. Estrogen

b. Progesterone

c. H.C.G

d. None of the above

198. Puerbral infection kis ka major cause hai?

a. PID

b. Puerperal sepsis

c. Septicaemia

d. Pyaemia

199. Puerperal sepsis ka commonest cause kiya hai?

a. Anaerobes

b. Gonococci

c Staphylococci

d. Streptococci

200. Tuwarad is a sign of:

a. Menarche

b. Menopause

c. Puberty

d. Climacterium

MD AMU ENTRANCE EXAMNATION
ANSWERS KEY 2006-07

1. B   2. D   3. C   4. C   5. B
6. C   7. D   8. B   9. B   10. D
11. B   12. B   13. D   14. A   15. D
16. D   17. C   18. C   19. B   20. B
21. B   22. B   23. C   24. B   25. B
26. B   27. D   28. B   29. C   30. C
31. C   32. C   33. C   34. A   35. C
36. D   37. A   38. B   39. D   40. C
41. D   42. B   43. C   44. A   45. D
46. B   47. D   48. D   49. B   50. A
51. B   52. D   53. C   54. B   55. D
56. D   57. B   58. A   59. B   60. A
61. D   62. C   63. D   64. B   65. C
66. C   67. B   68. A   69. A   70. D
71. D   72. B   73. D   74. A   75. D
76. D   77. B   78. A   79. A   80. D
81. C   82. D   83. D   84. C   85. D
86. B   87. A   88. D   89. C   90. A
91. C   92. D   93. D   94. C   95. D
96. C   97. D   98. A   99. D   100. A
101. A   102. B   103. C   104. D   105. B
106. A   107. D   108. A   109. A   110. C
111. A   112. B   113. A   114. C   115. B
116. C   117. C   118. A   119. A   120. B
121. C   122. A   123. A   124. A   125. D
126. C   127. A   128. C   129. D   130. B
131. D   132. D   133. A   134. A   135. C
136. B   137. A   138. B   139. B   140. C
141. B   142. D   143. D   144. A   145. B
146. A   147. D   148. B   149. B   150. D
151. C   152. C   153. D   154. A   155. D
156. C   157. C   158. B   159. B   160. C
161. D   162. A   163. D   164. B   165. B

166. A 167. D 168. D 169. B 170. B
171. B 172. D 173. A 174. C 175. B
176. B 177. D 178. D 179. C 180. C
181. A 182. A 183. C 184. B 185. A
186. D 187. C 188. B 189. A 190. D
191. B 192. A 193. B 194. B 195. A
196. B 197. C 198. C 199. D 200. B

1. Trench foot kin logon me hota hai:
a. Dhoop me kaam karne wale logon me
b. Cigrett pene wale logon me
c. Sardi me kaam karne wale logon me
d. None of the above

2. Courvoisiers law is related:
a. Jaundice
b. Uretric calculus
c. Fistula in ano
d. Portal hypertension

3. Kisi hadasha ke mareez me sab se pahle kis cheez ka khayal karna chhaiye:
a. Bleeding
b. Shock
c. Respiration
d. Voice

4. Sunflower cataract kis waja se hota hai:
a. Siderosis
b. Chalcosis
c. Pb intoxication
d. Silicosis

5. Darje zail anaesthetic dawao me qalb ke liye sab se kam muzir kan se dawa hai:
a. Erflurane
b. Isoflurane
c. Halothane
d. Trichloro ethelene

6. Jiryane khoon ko rokne wali Unani dawa:

a. Shahitarah

b. Barge neem

c. Ushba

d. None of the above

7. Longest acting anaesthesia is:

a. Bupvacaine

b. Tetracaine

c. Xylocaine

d. Cocaine

8. Sab se pahle local anaethesia ke liye kis dawa ka istemaal hoa:

a. Cocaine

b. Xylocaine

c. Lignocaine

d. Choloroform

9. Pahla local anaesthesia kis san me diya gaya

a. 1885

B. 1884

C. 1985

d. None of the above

10. Kis qism ke anaesthesia ke complication me mareez ko dard sar hota hai:

a. Local anaesthesia me

b. General anaesthesia me

c. Spinal anaesthesia me

d. All of the above

11. Ek mutthi barabar blood clot me kitna blood hota hai:

a. 250 ml

b. 300 ml

c. 450 ml
d. 500 ml

12. The normal length of cervix is:
a. 1.5 cm
b. 2.5 cm
c. 3.5 cm
d. 4 cm

13. Zonular cataract hai:
a. Bilateral
b. Stationary
c. Autosomal dominant
d. All

14. Most common position of fibroid is:
a. Intamural
b. Subserous
c. Submucous
d. Cervical

15. Aqueous humour ka afraz kis se hota hai:
a. Ciliary process
b. Iris
c. Lacrimal glands
d. Conjunctivitis

16.Waldeyers lymphatic ring me kaun sa gudad lymphavia shamil nahi hai:
a. Pharyngeal tonsil
b. Faucial tonsil
c. Abdominal tonsil
d. Lingual tonsil

17. Horners syndrome me hota hai:
a. Ectropion

b. Entropion

c. Trichiasis

d. Slight ptosis

18. Cortical cataract logon me amooman hota hai:

a. 20-25%

b. 30-40%

c. 50-65%

d. 75-80%

19. Cochlea ki shakal hoti hai:

a. Chand ki tarah

b. Seep ki tarah

c. Nao ki tarah

d. Ghonghe ki tarah

20. Sharpnells membrane kahte hai

a. Pars tensa ko

b. Fenestra vestibule ko

c. Pars flacida ko

d. Bowmans membrane

21. What is length of external auditory canal?

a. 12 mm

b. 24 mm

c. 8 mm

d. 16mm

22. Ye Stove in chest ki waja hai:

a. Double rib fracture

b. Single rib fracture

c. Steeting wheel injury

d. All of them

23. The most common bone tumors are:

a. Osteosarcoma

b.Osteoclastoma

c. Secondaries

d. Multiple myeloma

24. Renal calculi are seen in

a. Hyperthyroidism

b. Hyper parathyroidism

c. Cushings disease

d. Addisons disease

25. Most seriously affected organ in shock is:

a. Heart

b. Kidney

c. Liver

d. Spleen

26. Secondary hemorrhage occurs during:

a. 10-15 days after operation

b. 3-7 days keander

c. After 7-14 days after operation

d. All of the above

27. What percentage of of ovarian neoplasms are benign?

a. 10%

b. 30 %

c. 50 %

d. 75 %

28. Hospital dressing is best disposed of by:

a. Incineration

b. Dumping

c. Autoclaving

d. Burning

29. The most common malignancy seen in AIDS Patient is:

a. B- cell lymphoma

b. Burkitts lymphoma

c. Kaposi sarcoma

d. Leukaemia

30.Transfusion ke liye istemaal kiya jane wala khoon rakha jata hai:

a. $4\,C^0$

b. $1\,C^0$

c. $10\,C^0$

d. $6\,C^0$

31. Major surgery me post operative complication se maut waqai hoti hai:

a. Cardiac failure se

b. Severe hemorrhage se

c. Pulmonary embolism

d. Respiratory failure se

32. Women me paye jane wala inshaqae miqad hota hai:

a. Anterior fissure

b. Poterior fissure

c. Lateral wall fissure

d. None of the above

33. Universal tumor kahlata hai:

a. Lipoma

b. Sebaceous cyst

c. Neurofibroma

d. Leomeyoma

34. Iron is absorbed in:

a. Stomach

b. Duodenum

c. Jejinum

d. Colon

35. Which of the following tumor is associated with Meighs syndrome?

a. Fibroma ovary

b. Brenners tumor

c. Thecoma

d. All of the above

36. Turyris sign tashkhesi nishani hai:

a. Osteogenic carcinoma

b. Epilepsy

c. Meningitis

d. Sciatica

37. Tasamum boul waqai hota hai jabki GFR kam ho jaye:

a. 25 %

b. 50%

c. 60%

d. 80%

38. Parthes test kis uzu ki halat ko maloom karne ke liye istemaal me laya jata hai:

a. Deep arteries ko

b. Lymphatics channels ko

c. Bile duct ko

d. Deep veins ko

39. I.V.P me iodine ka kaun sa compound istemaal hota hai:
a. Inorganic iodine
b. Organic iodine
c. Radioactive iodine
d. Any of them

40. Chocolate cysts of ovary are seen in:
a. Endometriosis
b. Intracystic bleeding
c. Hemorrhagic follicular cyst
d. All of the above

41. Naram aur aapas me mile hoe ghudad lymphawia alamat hai:
a. Syphilis ki
b. Gonorrhoea ki
c. Hodgkins disease
d. Tuberculosis ki

42. Audible range of sound frequency:
a. 20-200 Hz
b. 20-2000 Hz
c. 20-200000 Hz
d. 20-2000 Hz

43. All are true about whooping cough except:
a. Bardetella purtusis is cause
b. Incubation period is 1-2 week

c. 1-2 week dry cough

d. Antibiotics are used for treatment

44. Sarsam ke ilaj me sab se pahle kiya karte hai:

a. Pashwia karte hain

b. Lakhlakha karte hai

c. Tabreed e ras karte hai

d. Huqna dete hain

45. Falghamoni aesa waram hai jo:

a. Khalis safra se paida hota hai

b. Khalis khoon se paida hota hai

c. Khalis balgham se paida hota hai

d. Khalis sauda se paida hota hai

46. Which of the following drug is used for prophylaxis of Leptospirosis?

a. Erythromycin

b. Ciprofloxacin

c. Doxycyclin

d. Sulfonamide

47. Streak ovaries are seen in:

a. Triple X syndrome

b. Turner syndrome

c. Kilinefilters syndrome

d. Down syndrome

48. Commonest type of gastric carcinoma of stomach:

a. Squamous cell carcinoma

b. Adeno carcinoma

c. Non Hodgkins lymphoma

d. Leiomyo sarcoma

49. Young adult me platelets ki tabai tadad hoa karti hai:
a. 45000-850000 mm^3

b. 5000-9000 mm^3

c. 4.5-5.5 million mm^3

d. 200000-400000 mm^3

50. Following are causes of true precious puberty except?
a. Hyperthyroidism

b. Albright syndrome

c. Intracranial tumor

d. Granulosa cell tumor

51. Normal pressure of nabz:
a. 15 mm of Hg

b. 25 mm of Hg

c. 4o mm of Hg

d. 90 mm of Hg

52. Boule ghasali alamat hai:
a. Sozak

b. Syphilis

c. Zaufe kuliya

d. All of them

53. Gule banafsha, maveez munaqqa, beikh kasni, badyaan, gaozaban nuskha hai:

a. Nuzaj balgham ka

b. Mulayyan Tabbah ka

c. Khalal shikam ka

d. Dafae Tip ka

54. Facial nerve ka nucleus kaha hota hai:

a. Mid brain

b. Pons

c. Medulla

d. Cerebellum

55. Dawae Turanjabeen ko kis tarah istemaal karana hota hai:

a. Tanha

b. Paani me josh dekar

c. Doodh me josh dekar

d. Abe afsharda anaar me josh dekar

56. Zoosantaria istalahan hai:

a. Sue hazm ko kahte hai

b. Khooni ishal ko kahte hai

c. Ishal zaifee ko kahte hai

d. Zurb wa khulfa ko kahte hain

57. Atherosclerosis kis artery me nahi hoti hai:

a. Radial artery

b. Internal Mammary artery

c. Both a and b

d. Cerebral artery

58. Corticospinal tract kis jagah hota hai:
a. Posterior limb of internal capsule
b. Anterior limb of internal capsule
c. Both a and b
d. Substantia nigra

59. Arqun nisaa:
a. Asabi marz hai
b. Azali marz hai
c. Mufasali marz hai
d. None of the above

60. Clinically ziyadah tar viral hepatitis kis qism ki hoti hai:
a. Mild
b. Moderate
c. Severe
d. Asymptomatic

61. Lung ki gas exchange unit kiya hai:
a. Terminal bronchiole
b. Acinus
c. Pneumocytes
d. Terminal lobule

62. Kazaz me daura ke baad azlaat:
a. Apni tabai halat par laut ate hai
b. Istarkhai ho jate hai
c. Azlaat ki tasanuji halat kisi qadar barqarar rahti hai
d. All of the above

63. Hurqatul boul kis marz me maujood nahi hota hai:

a. Sozak

b. Iltihabe masana

c. Qaroohe ahleel

d. Boul fil farash

64. Surkhubadah ka other name kiya hai:

a. Namal

b. Banatul Lail

c. Humrah

c. Jumarah

65. Marz sozak ka madda sozaki jab khoon me shamil ho jata hai to kiya paida karta hai:

a. Pyaemia

b. Hematuria

c. Hemorrhage

d. Anaemia

66. Humme Matbaqa wah bukhar hai jo…….ki ufoonat se paida hota hai:

a. Safara

b. Khoon

c. Balgham

d. Sauda

67. What is population day?

a. 11 July

b. 11 May

c. 11 Febuary

d. 11 June

68. LBW ka itilaaq kab honga:

a. Jab bawaqt paidaish bacche ka wazan 2 kg se kam ho

b. Jab bawaqt paidaish bacche ka wazan 2.25 kg se kam ho

c. Jab bawaqt paidaish bacche ka wazan 2.50 kg se kam ho

d. Jab bawaqt paidaish bacche ka wazan 3 kg se kam ho

69. Trunk ka surface area hota hai:

a. 50 %

b. 36 %

c, 18 %

d. 60 %

70. Goose sign kis taraf ishara karta hai:

a. Diphtheria ki taraf

b. Measles ki taraf

c. Gharqani ki taraf

d. Yellow fever ki taraf

71. Kis qism ki muzamin simmiyat A,B,C,D,E,F,G,H.I ke bayan kiya jata hai:

a. Mercurry

b. Antimony

c. Arsenic

d. Kuchla

72. Dribling of salivation maut ki yaqeeni alamat hoti hai:

a. Suffocation

b. Hanging

c. Drowning

d. Strangulation

73. Hundred day cough is known as:

a. Diphtheria

b. Chiken pox

c. Migraine

d. Pertusis

74. Agar aurat HIV positive hai to uske nauzaida bacche me darje zail vaccine me se kaun sa hai:

a. O.P.V

b. B.C.G

c. Anti hepatitis B vaccine

d. All of the above

75. The most common cause of vaginitis in adult is:

a. Gonococcous

b. Trichomonas

c. Candiada

d. Chemical

76. Aaram ki halat me insaan fee ghanta kitni carbon dioxide kharij karta hai:

a. 0.5 cft

b. 0.7 cft

c. 0.9 cft

d. 0.3 cft

77. Teeke lagan eke qaumi programme ke tahat 5-6years ki umr ke baccho ko kaun sa teeka lagna chhaiye:

a. BCG

b. OPV

c. Measles

d. D.T

78. Which of the following is contraceptive drug:

a. Gule mundi

b. Laai

c. Barge arosa

d. Maghz tukhm bakain

79. Acute PID is most often is due to:

a. Chlamydia

b. Mycoplasma

c. Streptococci

d. E. coli

80. Which of the following cancer is related with virus:

a. Breast cancer

b. Oral cancer

c. Lung cancer

d. Cancer of cervix

81. Hindustan me National Rural Health Mission ka aghaz kab hua:

a. 1975

b. 1985

c. 1995

d. 2005

82. Gonorrhoea affects the following sites except?

a. Vagina

b. Cervix

c. Urethra

d. Bartholins gland

83. Which mosquito is also known as Tiger mosquito?

a. Anopheles

b. Culex

c. Aedes

d. Mansonia

84. America me red cross ki baani aur pahli khatoon sadar kaun hoi?

a. Nightangle

b. Aegameda

c. Helari klinton

d. Kilara barton

85. Primary health centre ke tehat kinte mareezo ka ilaj mumkin hai:

a. 20, 000

b. 30, 000

c. 40, 000

d. 50, 000

86. 100 Din ki khansi kahlati hai

a. Small pox

b. Chicken pox

c. Measles

d. None

87. In India when family palaning programme is started:
a. 1950
b. 1951
c. 1952
d. 1953

88. Causative organism of Toxic Shock Syndrome is:
a. Sterpticoccus
b. Staphylococcus
c. Gonococcus
d. E. coli

89. Pelvic inflammatory disease ka sabab hota hai:
a. Klebsiella
b. N. Gonorrhoea
c. Candida
d. Mycobacterium Leprae

90. What is legal permission for MTP?
a. 12 weeks
b. 30 weeks
c. 20 weeks
d. 24 weeks

91. Most common cause of pyometra is:
a. Endometrial carcinoma
b. IUCD
c. Sterile endometritis
d. Infected hematometra

92. Commonest cause of neonatal death is:

a. Ishali amraz

b. Respiratory infection

c. Prematurity

d. Congenital disorder

93. Non-pragnant endometrium is infected only:

a. Chalamydia

b. Gonococcus

c. Staphylococcus

d. All of the above

94. What should be the amount of blood loss to define menorrhagia?

a. 750 ml

b. 80 ml

c. 150 ml

d. 200 ml

95. Drug of choice in anovulatory DUB is:

a. Danazol

b. Clomiphene

c. Bromocriptine

d. Estrogen

96. Irregular acyclical bleeding from uterus is referred to as:

a. Epimenorrhaea

b. Metrorrhagaea

c. Menorrhagaea

d. Menometrorrhagaea

97. TOC in congenital UV prolapsed is:

a. Fothergills operation

b. Le fort operation

c. Cervicopexy

d. Pessary treatment

98. Caput succedaneum valadat ke kitne dino baad ghaib ho jata hai:

a. 3-7 days

b. 2-10 days

c. 1-2 days

d. 3-4 days

99. Lanugo kise kahte hai:

a. Fine facial hair

b. Axillary hair

c. Fine pubic hair

d. Eye brow

100. Haultains surgery is ferformed for:

a. Procidentia

b. Elongated cervix

c. Cervical fibroid

d. Chronic inversions of uterus

101. Neural tube defects is caused due to deficiency of:

a. Pyridoxin

b. Folic acid

c. Thiamine

d. Iron

102. Cancer cervix ka sab se common maut ka sabab kiya hai:
a. Renal failure
b. Hemorrhage
c. Sepsis
d. Hepatic failure

103. Turners syndrome me kitne chromosome hote hai:
a. 45 XO
b. 46 XX
c. 44 XY
d. 47 XXY

104. Internal rotation of head occurs in:
a. Cervix
b. Pelvic brim
c. Pelvic floor
d. Introitus

105. Spermatogonium ko mature spermatozoa banana ke liye kitne din darker hite hai:
a. 30 days
b. 40 days
c. 60 days
d. 100 days

106. Falopian tube ke bilateral obstruction ke liye kaun sa infection sabab hai:
a. Gonorrhoea
b. Syphilis
c. AIDS

d. Qarha rakhu

107. Jananeen ki aswate qalb sab sepahle kis ne daryaft kiya:
a. Buqrat
b. Herophelus
c. Jalonoos
d. Abu Sahal Masihi

108. Graffian follicle ka rupture kab hota hai:
a. L.H Surge se kuchh pahle
b. L.H Surge ke fauran baad
c. L.H Surge ke f6 hours baad
d. L.H Surge 16-24 hours ke baad

109. Ek mukammal masheema ke ander kitni khoon ki mikdaar hoti hai:
a. 500 ML
b. 250 ML
c. 750 ML
d. 200 ML

110. Childrens me mirgi ko kis naam se jana jata hai:
a. Aqaalul itifal
b. Ummus sibyaan
c. Attasul attafal
d. Kaboos

111. Chid bearing age me Menorrhagia ka sab se common sabab hai:
a. Pelvic endometriosis
b. DUB

c. Fibroid

d. Adenomyosis

112. The main cause of haemorrhage after delivery:
a. Retained placenta

b. Insaqaqurreham

b. Insaqaqurnarakh

d. insaqaqurunq

113. Triangle of Kochs kaha paya jata hai:
a. Liver

b. Pancreas

c. Heart

d. Brain

114. Tihal ki damwi parwarish:
a. Spleenic vien Pulmonary artery, Hepatic artery

b. Spleenic Arery , Gastric artery, Hepatic artery

c. Spleenic artery , Spleenic vien, Hepatic artery

d. None of the above

115. Virchows lymphnodes are:
a. Left supraclavicular L. node

b. Right supraclavicular L. node

c. Axillary L. node

d. Media stinal lymph node

116. Proteins absorbed in Git in the form of:
a. Peptones

b. Polypeptides

c. Amino acid

d. Amino peptides

117. Total lung capacity is depends on:

a. Size of airways

b. Closing volume

c. Lung compliance

d. Residual volume

118. Unidirectional flow of impulse in nerve at:

a. Synapse

b. Axon

c. Dendrites

d. All of the above

119. Normal quantity of gastric fluids is:

a. 2500-3000 ml

b. 4000-5000 ml

c. 1200-1500 ml

d. 20-25 ml

120. Puerperium extends upto:

a. 2 weeks

b. 4 weeks

c. 6 weeks

d. 12 weeks

121. Orthopnoa is found in which disease?

a. TB

b. Asthma

c. MI

d. CCF

122. Milk secretion start:

a. In first trimester

b. Second trimester

c. In last trimester

d. None

123. The normal pancreatic fluid is:

a. 3000 ml

b. 3500 ml

c. 2000 ml

d. 1500 ml

124. Acetyl choline ke asar ki tadeel karta hai:

a. Morphine

b. Nicotine

c. Atropne

d. None

125. What should be weight of the fetus to be called an abortous:

a. Less than 300 gm

b. Less than 500 gm

c. Less than 1000 gm

d. Less than 1500 gm

126. Most of abortion occurs in:

a. First 8 weeks

b. F 8-16 weeks

c. 16-20 weeks

d. 20-28 weeks

127. Contents of adductor canal is:

a. Saphenus nerve

b. Femoral nerve

c. Profunda femoris artery

d. Profunda femoris vein

128. Aorta is bifurcate at the level of:

a. Xiphisternal level

b. Symphysis pubic

c. At the level of umbilicus

d. Below the umbilicus

129. The types of Tanasuli Saqoot are:

a. 2

b. 3

c. 4

d. 5

130. Laxity of Pouch of Douglas is called:

a. Cystocele

b. Enterocele

c. Rectocele

d. Urethrocele

131. Total bones of face are:

a. 20

b. 08

c. 10

d. 14

132. Which muscle is multipinnate?

a. Teres major

b. Deltoid

c. Serratus anterior

d. Rectonalis major

133. Left gastroepiploic artery kis ki branch hai

a. Spleenic artery

b. Coelic artery

c. Hepatic artery

d.Superior mesenteric artery

134. Which statement is correct about Zenkers diverticulum?

a. Asymptomatic hota hai

b. Oesophagus ke darmiyaan me hota hai

c. Sigmoid colon ke pass hota hai

d. Childrens me hota hai

135. Kis marz me siyah qarura bura hai?

a. Amraz Kabid

b. Amraz Tihal

c. Amraz Qalb

d. Amraz Kulya wa Masana

136. Ghee ki tarah sufaid qarurah ko kehte hain:

a. Mukhati

b. Dasmi

c. Ihali

d. Nuqai

137. Marz muzmin me Gurdon me bol hota hai:

a. Jhag der tak rehta hai

b. Jhag jald tut jata hai

c. Jhag zyada na paida hote hain

d. Jhag kam paida hote hain

138. Hormones are found in

a. Jalapa

b. Jund baidaster

c. Beejband

d. Qeemoliya

139. Qaimunnar kiya jata hai:

a. Garbh jantar

b. Jal jantar

c. Pataal jantar

d. Damro jantar

140. Safoofe tihal me ziyadah tar mustamil hai:

a. Namkiyat

b. Tukhmiyat

c. Haleela jat

d. Sheerajat

141. Kushta mussala ke ajza hai:

a. Qalai, para, raskapoor

b. Qalai, gaudanti, marjaan

c. Qalai, jasta, seesa

d. Qalai, hartal, tootiya

142. Atees ko kis Tibb se hasil kiya gaya hai:

a. Allopathic

b. Homeopath

c. Ayurvadh

d. Unani

143. Gramophon ke record se banaya jata hai:
a. Katerra
b. Kath
c. Murr
d. Luk

144. Word drug kis zubaan se makhooz hai:
a. Unani
b. Latin
c. Qadeem mishri
d. English

145. Which drug is reaches to fetus through placenta:
a. Insulin
b. Narcotics
c. Habbul qilqil
d. Qurs zaheer

146. Nabeez kiya hai:
a. Ghair muqatar sharab
b. Tukhm kezariye taiyar kiya hoa murakkab
c. Dawao ka khesandah
d. Dawao ka joshanda

147. Bol Karafsi ka rang hota hai?
a. Sufaid sabzi mayal
b. Zardi mayal khaki
c. Zardi mayal surkh
d.Sufaid zardi mayal

148. Bol Rusub Makhati is a diagnosis of?

a. Nazj mawad

b. Ghalba balgham

c. Khilt ghaliz wa kham

d. A, B & C

149. Maaul Hayat kahte hai

a. Shahad, Suhaga, Ghee

b. Suhaga, Ghee

c. Shahad , Ghee, Egg

d. None

150. The nabz of Zatur Riah:

a. Nabz Mouji

b. Nabz Manshari

c. Nabz Mamtali

d. Nabz Mukhtalif

151. The nabz of Ghib Daira:

a. Nabz Munkhafiz, Sagheer wa Mutfawut

b. Nabz Munkhafiz, Sagheer wa Mukhtalif

c. Nabz Munkhafiz, Sagheer wa Mutawatir

d. Nabz Munkhafiz, Sagheer wa Mamtali

152. The nabz of Subat:

a. Nabz Sulb

b. Nabz Mukhtalif

c. Nabz Sagheer

d. Nabz Mamtali

153. Cod liver oil is obtained from:

a. From Gadus morrhua

b. From Gallus domesticus

c. From Hirundo medicinalis

d. From Coccus lacca

154. The author of 'Kitabul Ahwia wal Miyah' is:

a. Buqrat

b. Jalinoos

c. Razi

d. Ibn Sina

155. Which type of water causes Pseudopregnancy:

a. Mae Matriya

b. Mae Naz

c. Mae Saljiya

d. Mae Rakid

156 . For preservation of murakkabat drug which is used:

a. Tartaric acid

b. Benzene

c. Benzoic acid

d. Sodium benzoate

157. Ilmul Advia kitne mazaameen par mustamil hai:

a. 2

b. 3

c. 4

d. 5

158. Sankhia and para ka murakkab hai:

a. Darchini

b. Darhald

c. Raskapoor

d. Darchikna

159. Dawa ke sab se lateef ajza ko kiya kahte hai:

a. Rakhu mutlaq

b. Rakhu bafraat

c. Rakhu jidan

d. Rakhu lateef

160. Fayil bil Johar hota hai

a. Jo apni kaifiyat se asar kare

b. Jo apne madde se asar kare

c. Jo apni surat nuiya se asar kare

d. All of the above

161. Agar dakhil shuda chezen badan ke mushaba na hon:

a. Ghiza Mutlaq kehte hain

b. Dawae Mutlaq kehte hain

c. Dawae Ghizai kehte hain

d. Dawae Motadil kehte hain

162. Fatty foods are

a. Giza Kaseef Kaseerul Taghzia

b. Giza Kaseef Qaleelul Taghzia

c. Giza Kaseef Kaseerul Taghzia Jayadul Kimus

d. Giza Kaseef Kaseerul Taghzia Raddiul Kimus

163. Death caused due to good news is termed as:
a. Sadma
b. Shadi Nagahani
c. Marg Nagahani
d. Shadi Marg

164. The Rooh gushes towards outwards slowly during:
a. Anger
b. Joy
c. Fear
d. Sorrow

165. The sabab of Ikhtilaj is:
a. Kasrat Yabusat
b. Kasrat Burudat
c. Kasrat Riyah
d. Kasrat Fuzlat

166. Nail bed of thumb is supplied by
a. Radial Nerve
b. Ulnar Nerve
c. Median Nerve
d. None of the above

167. Halocrine secretion is seen in .... gland
a. Salivary
b.Mammary
c. Sebaceous
d. Gastric

168. All have no lymphatics, except

a. Brain

b. Internal ear

c. Dermis

d. Eye

169. Muscles of tongue supplied by

a. Linguinal Nerve

b. Glossopharyngeal Nerve

c. Chorda tympani

d. Hypoglossal

170. Cowper's glands open into:

a. Prostatic urethra

b. Membranous urethra

c. Penile urethra

d. Bulbar urethra

171. First carpometacarpal joint is a:

a. Hinge joint

b. Saddle joint

c. Elipsoid joint

d. Synovial joint

172. The nerve supply to pronator teres:

a. Median Nerve

b. Radial Nerve

c. Ulnar Nerve

d. Posterior Interosseous Nerve

173. Slpenic artery supplies the following, except:

a. Liver

b. Pancreas

c. Spleen

d. Stomach

174. Action of quadrator femoris is:

a. Flexion

b. Extension

c. Lateral rotation

d. Medial rotation

175. Bile duct opens into:

a. Second part of Duodenum

b. Third part of Duodenum

c. Pyloric end of stomach

d. Ileo-caecal junction

176. Negri bodies kaha payi jati hai:

a. Hippocampus

b. Mid brain

c. Basal ganglion

d. Posterior cortex

177. Langehans cells kis tarah ke hote hai:

a. Phagocytic

b. Antigen presenting nature

c. Anti immune nature

d. None of the above

178. Jarasheem ka dakhli zahar kahlata hai:

a. Nephrotoxin

b. Neurotoxin

c. Endotoxin

d. Exotoxin

179. Cloudy degeneration kahlata hai:

a. Albuminous

b. Protenous

c. Carbohydrates

d. Fats

180. Istiwa wa ikhtilaf kis se mansoob hai:

a. Nabz khali se

b. Nabz sulb se

c. Nabz har se

d. Nabz mustawi se

181. Imshaaje badan kiya hai:

a. Akhlat

b. Johare aaza

c. Madda e manawia

d. Sheer mader

182. Raha kis ko kahte hai:

a. Us garhe ko jo hateli me hota hai

b. Us garhe ko jo qalb me hota hai

c. Ek ratoobat ko

d. Ek aqleem ko

183. Mandarja zail asbab baroodat paida karte hai except?

a. Ehtabas wa istifragh ki ziyadti

b. Sukoon wa neend ki ziyadti

c. Ghiza me kami

d. Ufoonat ka hona

184. Miqdaar ke lihaz se nabz ki qisme hain except?

a. Taweel, areez. Munkhafis

b. Kasir, zeeq, motadil

c. Taweel, zeeq, saree

d. Taweel, zeeq, kasir, zeeq

185. Toughest layer in Esophagus is:

a. Mucosa

b. Submucosa

c. Muscularis

d.Adventia

186. Post mortem staining' is termed as:

a. Cadaver lividity

b. Hypostasis

c. Suggligations

d. All

187. Commonest organ to be injured in bomb blast is:

a. Liver

b. Lung

c. Skin

d. Spleen

188. The IPC act associated with grievous injury is:

a. 300

b. 304A

c. 320

d.302

189. Hydrocution is:

a. Electrocution in water

b. Dry drowning

c. Drowning in cold water

d. Post mortem immersion

190. Gettler 's test is used to diagnose death due to:

a. Drowning

b. Hanging

c. Burns

d. Phosphorus poisoning

191. Hyoid fracture is common in:

a. Hanging

b. Stangulation

c. Throttling

d. Chocking

192. A sample to look for uric acid crystals would be submitted to lab in:

a. Formalin

b. Alcohol

c. Distilled water

d. Normal saline

193. Smell of bitter almonds is perceived in poisoning with:
a. Phosphorus
b. Hydrocyanic acid
c. Nitric acid
d. Oxalic acid

194. Preservative used for toxicological specimen:
a. 20% formalin
b. Saturated sodium chloride
c. 20% alcohol
d. 10% alcohol

195. Gastric levage can be done in poisoning with:
a. Carbolic acid
b. Oxalic acid
c. Sulphuric acid
d. Caustic potash & soda

196. Fatal period of Sulphuric acid poisoning is:
a. 2-4 hrs
b. 6-10 hrs
c. 12-16 hrs
d. 8-14 hrs

197. The poison that can be detected in hair, long after death is:
a. Lead
b. Mercury
c. Arsenic
d. Cannabis

198. Mercury poison acts on:

a. Proximal convoluted tubule

b. Distal convoluted tubule

c. Loope of Henle

d. Collecting ducts

199. Erethism occurs in:

a. Hg

b. As

c. Pb

d. Cu

200. Reinsch's test is used for detection of:

a. Arsenic

b. Lead

c. Strychnine

d. Mercury

MD AMU ENTRANCE EXAMNATION
ANSWERS KEY 2005-06

1. C   2. A   3. C   4. B   5. C
6. D   7. A   8. A   9. B   10. C
11. D   12. B   13. D   14. A   15. A
16. C   17. D   18. D   19. D   20. C
21. C   22. A   23. A   24. B   25. A
26. C   27. D   28. A   29. C   30. A
31. B   32. B   33. A   34. B   35. B
36. A   37. A   38. D   39. C   40. A
41. C   42. B   43. C   44. D   45. B
46. C   47. A   48. B   49. C   50. D
51. A   52. C   53. C   54. B   55. C
56. B   57. B   58. A   59. A   60. D
61. B   62. C   63. D   64. C   65. A
66. B   67. A   68. C   69. B   70. C
71. B   72. B   73. D   74. A   75. B
76. B   77. D   78. B   79. A   80. D
81. D   82. A   83. C   84. C   85. B
86. D   87. C   88. B   89. B   90. C
91. D   92. C   93. B   94. B   95. B
96. B   97. C   98. C   99. A   100. D
101. B   102. A   103. A   104. C   105. C
106. A   107. C   108. D   109. A   110. B
111. B   112. A   113. C   114. B   115. A
116. C   117. C   118. A   119. C   120. C
121. D   122. A   123. D   124. C   125. B
126. A   127. B   128. D   129. D   130. B
131. D   132. B   133. A   134. B   135. D
136. C   137. A   138. B   139. B   140. A
141. C   142. C   143. D   144. D   145. A
146. A   147. B   148. C   149. A   150. A
151. B   152. D   153. A   154. A   155. D
156. D   157. C   158. D   159. B   160. C
161. D   162. B   163. D   164. C   165. C

166. C 167. C 168.A 169. D 170. C
171. B 172. A 173. A 174. B 175. A
176. A 177. A 178. C 179. A 180. D
181. C 182. A 183. D 184. C 185. C
186. D 187. A 188 . C 189. C 190. A
191. C 192. B 193. B 194. B 195. A
196. C 197. C 198. A 199. A 200. A

1. In arthritis which cardiac valve is affected:
a. Mitral valve
b. Tricuspid valve
c. Aortic valve
d. Pulmonary valve

2. Khibta kis qism ka sudaa hai:
a. Sudaee har
b. Sudaee barid kharji
c. Sudaee damwi
d. Sudaee safrawi

3. Atibba Qurse afsanteen aur habbe karanjawa ka istemaal batoor e:
a. Qabz karte hain
b. Mushil karte hain
c. Dafae humma karte hain
d. Muqawwe bah karte hain

4. Nabz minshari payi jati hai:
a. Warme dimagh me
b. Warme qalb me
c. Warme ghishaur riya me
d. Warme aghshia me

5. Nabz munkhafis wah nabz hai:
a. Bulandi me motadil se kam ho
b. Bulandi me motadil se kam ho
c. Chauri me motadil se ziyadah ho
d. Chauri me motadil se kam ho

6. Zauf e Tihal me mufeed hai:
a. Barge gaozabah

b. Barge jhao
c. Barge karam kalla
d. Barge banafsha

7. Influenza dar haqeeqat hai:
a. Nzal haa
b. Nazla wabai barid
c. Nazla wabai har
d. Nazla barid

8. Khunaaq kis uzu ka marz hai:
a. Lauztain
b. Reham
c. Ghuddah nakfia
d. Halaq

9. Rag e Qeefal oayi jati hai:
a. Kohni ke jor ke qareeb bairoono janib
b. Kohni ke jor ke qareeb andarooni janib
c. Takhna ke jor ke qareeb bairoono janib
d. Takhna ke jor ke qareeb bairoono janib

10. Babinkis sign aam taur par paya jata hai:
a. Lower motor neuron disorder
b. Upper motor neuron disorder
c. Mixed neyron disordered
d. All of the above

11. Zoosantariya damwi me jiryanuddam ho sakta hai:
a. Large intestine
b. Small intestine
c. Both of theabove
d. None of the above

12. Nabz multavi (Delayed pulse) sabab hoa karti hai:
a. Atherosclerosis ki
b. Aortic stenosis ki

c. Thyrotixicosis ki

d. Co-arctation of aorta ki

13. Zaeeful amal aur mustarakun nafa Advia ka nuskha kaun sa hai:

a. Nuskha khalal shikam

b. Nuskha maul usool

c. Nuskha munzij balgham

d. Maaul usl

14. Amraze chasm par kis ki tasneef hai:

a. Abusahal masihi ki

b. Hanain bin ishaq

c. Alauddin

d. Ibne nafis

15. Bawaseer damia me pahle kiya kharij hota hai:

a. Khoon wa baraz mila hoa

b. Mukhat wa baraz mila hoa

c. Baraz

d. Khoon

16. Ghashi ki soorat me nabz kaisi hoti hai?

a. Qawwi

b. Mumtali

c. Minshari

d. Zaeef

17. Quwwate mukhayala ka muqam hai:

a. Muqaddam dimagh

b. Wast dimagh

c. Mokhar dimagh

d. Total dimagh

18. Kimiyawi taur par poodina ko kahte hai:

a. Menthol

b. Camphor
c. Thymol
d. Oil of peppermint

19. Habbul saudaa darasal hai:
a. Kala dana
b. Zeera siyah
c. Kalunji
d. Habbul qilqil

20. Juzam ke liye ek Unani mufarad dawa hai:
a. Olive oil
b. Turmeric oil
c. Chalmoora oil
d. Almond oil

21. Inzeer ka nabati name:
a. Ficus carica
b. Ficus racemosa
c. Ficus indica
d. Ficus religiosa

22. Qurse mussalas me shamil teen khubodar dawai hai:
a. Mushk, amber, zafran
b. Mushk, sandal, zafran
c. Sandal amber, zafran
d. Sandal, Kafoor zafran

23. Emulsion ki mishal par nishan lagaye:
a. Oil and water
b. Sirka and honey
c. Namak aur pani
d. Sirka and water

24. Majoon falasfa ka nafa khas:
a. Tanweem
b. Taskeen
c. Taqwiyate dimagh
d. Taqwiyate qalb

25. Which of the following drug is not an antibiotic?
a. Phenoxy methylpenicillin
b. Amoxycillin
c. Ciprofloxacin
d. Paracetamol

26. Which of the following drug is not plant origin?
a. Morphine
b. Reserpine
c. Ajmaline
d. Pentazocin

27. Which vitamin is water soluble?
a. Vitamin A
b. Vitamin C
c. Vitamin D
d. Vitamin K

28. Which drug is an antidote?
a. Narkachoor
b. Jadwar
c. Kuchla
d. Zaravand

29. Qanbeel ka other name:
a. Kalaunji
b. Kameela
c. Marchoba
d. Beikh hayat

30. Nausader ka shumaar kis me hai?
a. Zuel arwah
b. Zuel ijad wa arwah
c. None of the above
d. Zuel nafoos

31. Ismaaul Advia kis ki Tasneef hai:
a. Sharif khan
b. Aazam khan
c. Razi
d. Ibne baitar

32. Nabati dawa par nishan lagaye:
a. Abresham
b. Jawakhar
c. Hiran khuri
d. Jund baidaster

33. Hazar dana ki kiya mahiyat hai:
a. Bulbul
b. Nabat
c. Fakhta
d. Mitti

34. That drug which contain maximum potassium content:
a. Badam
b. Olive oil
c. Makhan
d. Cheeni

35. Quwwate nafsnia ka markazi organ hai:
a. Brain
b. Spinalcord
c. Nerves
d. Liver

36. Khilt ke laghwi meaning kiya hai?
a. Liquid things
b. Mixed things
c. Gaseous thins
d. Solid things

37. According to Ibne Sina kaha ke basined ziyadah motadil hote hai?
a. Qutub sumali
b. Khate saratn
c. Khate jiddi
d. Khate istiwa

38. Organs ka shumar kis me hota hai?
a . Arkane arba
b. Asbabe sitta zarooriya
c. Umoore Tabaiya
d. Quwwa

39. Kis hazam ke baad ghiza is qabil hoti hai ki tamaam aaza ko ghiza faraham ho sake:
a. Hazme medi
b. Hazme kabidi
c. Hazme urooqi
d. Hazme uzwi

40. Most reliable method of identification of a persion is by:
a. Fingerprinting
b. DNA Analysis
c. Scars
d. Anthrapometry

41. Darje zail ki kaun se tarkeeb ghalat hai:
a. Har yabis
b. Barid yabis

c. Har ratab
d. Ratab yabis

42. Mirarah se safra ka insabab kaha hota hai:
a. Liver
b. Duodenum
c. Mari
d. Ileum

43. Sabab:
a. Bizaat muqadam hota hai
b. Bizaat mokhar hota hai
c. Bizaat moasar hota hai
d. None of the above

44. Sange gurdah ki alamat kiya hai:
a. Boule tabani
b. Qiwame Aala
c. Rasoobe rimli
d. Yaqza

45. Kis sin ka mizaj motadil tareen hai:
a. Sine namu
b. Sine shabab
c. Sine kaholat
d. Sine saikhokhat

46. Hakeem Ajmal Khan ka intiqaal kaha hoa?
a. Delhi me
b. Rampur
c. Hyderabad
d. Aligarh

47. Arkan wah baseet ijsaam hai jo insaan ke ajzae awalia hain:
a. Buqrat ki

b. Zakaria razi ki

c. Hakeem sayyad istiyaque ahmar ki

d. Ibne Sina

48. Qaroora me rasoobb ki miqdaar hogi:

a. Masame garama me

b. Masame sard me

c. Masame khareef me

d. Masame rabee me

49. Qalb ke zariyah istemaal ki jane wali rooh ka intalaq hota hai:

a. Roohe nafsani

b. Roohe haiwani

c. Roohe tabaiya

d. None of the above

50. Naume yaqza ek qism hai:

a. Istifragh ki

b. Ehtabas ki

c. Asbabe zarooriya

d. Asbabe ghair zarooriya

51. Safara intestine me gir kar hazm karta hai:

a. Fats ko

b. Vitamin ko

c. Madiniyat ko

d. All of the above

52. Vascular pannus kis marz me paya jata hai:

a. Trachoma

b. Glaucoma

c. Cataracat

d. Vitamin A deficiency

53. Tibb ka babe Aadm kise mana jata hai:

a. Galen

b. Hippocrates

c. Rhazes

d. Ibne Sina

54. Hydophobia in me se kis bimaari ko kahte hai:
a. Cholera

b. Viral hepatitis

c. Rabies

d. Heat stroke

55. Who is known as pioneer of experimental medicine?
a. Hakeem Mohammad Ajmal Khan

b. Zakaria Razi

c. Jalinoos

d. Abul Qasim Zohravi

56. Rabies can be transmitted by all of the following except?
a. Bites

b. Licks

c. Aerosol

d. Ingestion

57. WHO ko kitne ilaqo me taqseem kiya gaya hai?
a. 10

b. 5

c. 6

d. 4

58. Huang Ti kis Tibb ka shanshanh kahlata hai:
a. Tibatti Tibb

b. Chini Tibb

c. Babli Tibb

d. Srelankai Tibb

59. National programme for the control of blindness is called:
a. Vision 2020
b. Vision 1999
c. Vision 1919
d. Vision 2000

60. Two years children me upper jaw me teeth kitne hote hai?
a. 12
b. 22
c. 10
d. 32

61. Gastroenteritis is a food born disease infected by?
a. Bacteria
b. Viral
c. Parasites
d. None of the above

62. What is infectious agent of Sars Disease?
a. Sabia virus
b. H5N1
c. Nipha virus
d. Corona virus

63. WHO ka head quarte kaha hai?
a. Newyork
b. Alma atta
c. New Delhi
d. Geneva

64. Kiya sahi hai jo mustamil hai?
a. Hifzane sehat
b. Tahaffuzi sehat

c. Tahaffuzi Tibb
d. Tibb Muhafizi

65. Aaz taleem sehat ke kliye ziyadah zaroori hai:
a. Nazla zukam ke liye
b. AIDS ke liye
c. Fracture ke liye
d. Dance ke liye

66. Sooraj ki roshni kis Vitamin ko banati hai:
a. Vtamin A
b. Vtamin D
c. Vtamin C
d. Vtamin E

67. Which of the following is nota feature of Patersion-Kelly (Plummer-Vinsion) syndrome?
a. Glossitis
b. Anaemia
c. Dysphagia
d. Clubbing of Finger

68. Rules of halves ka relation kis disease se hai?
a. Coronary heart disease
b. Hypertension
c. DM
d. Stroke

69. Female genital tract me Tubercular infection sabse ziyadah common kaha hai:
a. Uterus
b. Fallopian Tube
c. Ovaries
d. Endometrium

70. Littres Hernia is associated with which?
a. Circumference of the intestine
b. W shaped two loops of small intestine
c. Meckels diverticulum
d. None of the above

71. Albinism is caused by which enzyme deficiency?
a. Albinism
b. Tyrisinase
c. Tryponium
d. None

72. Spermatogonium ko mature spermatozoa banana ke liye kitne din lagte hai?
a. 30 days
b. 60 days
c. 90 days
d. 120 days

73. Daaul Feel Furj ke asbab hain:
a. Syphilis
b. Diq
c. Failaria
d. All of the above

74. Secondary renal calculi are generally composed of:
a. Calcium oxalate
b. Uric acid and urates
c. Cystine
d. Calcium ammonium magnesium phosphate

75. Which of the following is main cause of death in cervical cancer?
a. Severe weakness due to cancer
b. Bleeding
c. Uraemia

d. Bowel obstruction

76. Uterine hyper stimulation due to?
a. Oxyticics
b. Oxytocin
c. Prostaglandin
d. A.C.T.H

77. Gonorrhoea ka naam kis ne diya?
a. Galen
b. Hippocrates
c. Leuvon Hock
d. Neisser

78. Which of the following is correct for direct hernia?
a. Its descends obliquely downwards and medially
b. Impulse on coughing is felt on index fnger
c. It reduces when the patient lies down
d. All of the above

79. Muhafiz jananeen drugs me kaun se drug shamil nahi hai?
a. Khameera Murvareed
b. Tiryaqe Farooq
c. Daaul misk
d. Lauq khiyar shambar

80. Mc Burneys point lies along the line joining the anterior superior iliac spine and umbilicus at the junction of:
a. Medial $1/3^{rd}$ and lateral $2/3^{rd}$
b. Medial $2/3^{rd}$ and lateral $1/3^{rd}$
c. Medial 1/2 and lateral 2/2
d. Medial $3/4^{th}$ and lateral $1/4^{th}$

81. TORCH TEST mandarja zail kisi ek ki beemari ki nishandahi nahi karta hai is par nishaan lagon:
a. Toxoplasmosis
b. Rabies
c. CMV
d. Herpes simplex type II

82. Episiotomy structure cut is:
a. Anterior vaginal wall
b. Bulbospongiosus and parital of levator ani
c. Pudendal arteries
d. Lateral deep perineal muscles

83. Which of the following book is not written by Buqrat?
a. Kitabul Ajana
b. Kitabul aujaul Nisaa
c. Kitabul jananeen
d. Firdosul Hikmat

84. Failure of fusion of mullerian ducts may lead to formation of which uterus?
a. Arcuate
b. Bicornuate
c. Septate
d. All of the above

85. Zakhm ka accha na hona mandarja zail me se kis asar andaz nahi hota hai?
a. Umr
b. Jins
c. Yarqaan
d. Ghiza

86. Koun sa paidaishi sinus hai?
a. Periaurucular sinus
b. Plonidal sinus

c. Median mental sinus

d. None of the above

87. Length of common bile duct is:
a. 2.5 cm

b. 3.5 cm

c. 5.5 cm

d. 7.5 cm

88. Deep inguinal ring paya jata hai:
a. 1.5 cm above mid paint of inguinal ligament

b. 25 cmabove the pubic tubercle

c. None of the above

d. 2.5 cm above the mid inguinal ligament

89. Blood loss me koun se nishani nahi payi jati hai:
a. Nabz ka rafter ka tez hona

b. Becheni ka barhana

c. B.P ka increase hona

d. Urine ka kam hona

90. Kitabul Tasreef ka musanif koun hai:
a. Ibne Sina

b. Abu bakar Zakaria Rhaze

c. Abul Qasim Zohrawi

d. Ibne quf

91. Which vitamin is necessary for wound healing?
a. Vitamin D

b. Vitamin A

c. Vitamin C

d. Vitamin H

92. Actinomycosis ki sabse aam qism hai?
a. Facio cervical

b. Thoracic

c. Abdomen

d. Leg

93. What are the sign and symptoms of Tetanus?
a. Tetanus toxoids se

b. Exotoxin of Ch. Tetani se

c.. Exotoxin fixed to motor se

d. Dard ki waja se

94. Ulcer ki biopsy ke liye munasib hai:
a. Centre of ulcer

b. Edge of ulcer

c. Edge of ulcer along with some normal tissue

d. Base of the ulcer

95. Cause of delayed puberty:
a. Hypogonadotrophic Hypogonadism

b. Prostag;andin

c. Oxytocin

d. Non of the above

96. Curling ulcer paya jata hai:
a. On face

b. In fingers

c. On nose

d. In stomach

97. Nasolacrimal duct kaha khulti hai:
a. Superior meatus

b. Middle meatus

c. Inferir meatus

d. None of the above

98. Pseudomeigis syndrome is:
a. Ascites + Right hydrothorax

b. Ascites + Left hydrothorax

c. Ascites + Right hydrothorax + Fibroma

d. Ascites + Left hydrothorax + Fibroma

99. Cocks peculiar tumor kiya hota hai:

a. Papilloma

b. Squamous cell carcinoma

c. Osteomyelitis of scalp

d. Infected sebaceous cyst of scalp

100. Kaha ke stich jaldi kate jate hai?

a. Face

b. Chest

c. Abdomen

d. Perineum

101. In ascites shifting dullness is found if fluid accumulation becomes:

a. 100 ml

b. 200 ml

c. 300 ml

d. 500 ml

102. Mandibular nerve is the branch of:

a. Trigeminal nerve

b. Facial nerve

c. Abducent nerve

d. Trochlear nerve

103. Angle of the mandible ke gird asabi parwarish kis asaab ke zariye hoti hai?

a. Greater auricular

b. Lener occipital

c. Greater occipital

d. Trochlear nerve

104. Jigar se venous blood, IVC me kis vareed ke zariye ata hai?
a. Portal vein
b. Hepatic vein
c. Superior mesenteric vein
d. Inferior mesenteric vein

105. Mufasil bainul salmiyat inter phalangeal kis qism ka hai?
a. Pivot
b. Suture
c. Ball and socket
d. Condylar

106. Deep inguinal ring is me maujood rahti hai:
a. Transversus abdominis
b. Fascia transversalis
c. External oblique abdominis
d. Internal oblique abdominis

107. IVC ka empression hota hai:
a. Left lung
b. Right lung
c. Spleen
d. Pancreas

108. Jism ka sabse lamba azla hai:
a. Psoas major
b. Pectoralis major
c. Sartorius
d. Risorius

109. End organ of hearing kahte hai:
a. Tympanic membrane
b. Modeolus
c. Organ of corti

d. Stapes bone

110. In portal hypertension which clinical features is absent?
a. Spleenomegaly
b. Hematemesis and Malena
c. Ascites
d. None

111. Dimagh me abscess kis muqaam par hota hai?
a. Frontal lobe
b. Occipital lobe
c. Parital lobe
d. Temporal lobe

112. In fallots tetralogy which symptoms is not present in this disease:
a. V.S,D
b. Infundibular pulmonary stenosis
c. Overriding of aorta
d. Left ventricular hypertrophy

113. The commonest site of gastric carcinoma:
a. Lesser curvature
b. Greater curvature
c. Pylorus
d. None of the above

114. Testicular biopsy karana bahtar hai:
a. In azoospermia
b. In oligospermia
c. In polyspermia
d. Necrospermai

115. Diabetic retinopathy ke mareez me achanak basarat ke zaail hone ka sabab hai:
a. Papilloedema
b. Glaucoma
c. Cataract
d. Victreous haemorrhage

116. Spleenectomy sabse ziyadah bahtar hai:
a. Sickle cell anaemia
b. Hereditory spherocytosis
c. Thallassaemia
d. Non hodgkins lymphoma

117. Bawaseer damia me kaisa khoon kharij hota hai:
a. Munjamid
b. Sayyal
c. Siyah
d. Tazah sayyal surkh rang ka

118. Study of cancer is:
a. Brachiopathy
b. Cancerology
c. Oncology
d. Sistology

119. Uterus ke nikalne kea mal ko kiya kahte hai?
a. Uterine surgery
b. Hystrectomy
c. Uterus surgery
d. All of the above

120. Translumination test ziyadah karaamadh sabit hota hai:
a. Frontal sinusitis
b. Ethamoidal sinusitis
c. Sphenoidal sinusitis

d. Maxillary sinusitis

121. Rheumatic fever is manifested by:
a. Arthritis and carditis
b. Chorea
c. Erythema marginatum and subcutaneous nodules
d. All of the above

122. Rodent ulcer aam taur par kaha paida hota hai:
a. Limb
b. Face
c. Abdomen
d. Trunk

123. Roohe nafsani ka markaz hai:
a. Dimagh
b. Qalb
c. Kabid
d. Riya

124. Kisi uzu ki tabiyat maaloom karne ke liye kin umoor ko paishnazar rakha jata hai:
a. Mizaj ko
b. Sakht ko
c. Quwwat wa fail ko
d. All of the above

125. Mosam khareef kahte hai:
a. Mosame bahar ko
b. Mosame Khazan ko
c. Mosame barsaat ko
d. Mosame sarma ko

126. Elaam us amal ko kahte hai jis me:
a. Dard wa lazah paida kiya jaye
b. Dard wa lazah kam kiya jaye

c. Dard wa lazah khatm kiya jaye

d. All of the above

127. Ibne Sina ke according alwane boul:

a.18

b. 5

c. 6

d. 7

128. Rasoobe boul ghair tabai ke aqsaam:

a. 12

b. 8

c. 14

d. 11

129. Ilme kemiyah ki daryaft ke mutabiq quarti anasir ke tadad:

a. 106

b. 95

c. 92

d. 96

130. Jab safra raqeeq balgham ke sath mil jata hai to kiya kahlata hai?

a. Safra zinjari

b. Safra mirrah

c. Safra kurasi

d. Safra muhayya

131. Jab maddah kisi uzuerais se muntaqil ho kar adna uzu ki taraf ata hai:

a. Intaqale jayyad

b. Intaqale Aala

c. Intaqale Adna

d. Intaqale Raddi

132. Naseem par rooh ka itilaaq kab hota hai:
a. Jab wah bairooni hawa se juada ho jaye
b. Jab wah hunzarah me pahuch jaye
c. Jab wah Riya me pahuch jaye
d. Jab wah khoon me shamil hi jaye

133. Ratoobate Talayya ka shumar kis me hota hai:
a. Ratoobate ain
b. Ratoobate lymphawia
c. Ratoobate Oola
d. Ratoobate sani

134. Thermoregulatory centre is present in:
a. Frontal brain
b. Hind brain
c. Hypothalamus
d. M.O

135. Muscles fatigues ki waja bataiye:
a. Acetyl choline
b. Uric acid
c. Pyuric acid
d. Lactic acid

136. Which hormone increase the heart rate and B.P?
a. Pitutarian
b. Testosterone
c. Progesterone
d. Adrenaline

137. Which enzyme of tear is a germicide?
a. Lysozyme
b. Hysozyme
c. Occulozyme
d. Protozyme

138. Darje zail me se koun juzj blood brain barrier ko cross nahi karta hai:
a. Glucose
b. Insulin
c. Urea
d. Testosterone

139. A.D.H Gurde ke darje zail tammam me se kis muqamam par asar andaz hota hai:
a. Loop of Henle
b. Collecting duct
c. Vasa rectae
d. PCT

140. Neuro muscular junctions par neuro transmitter kiya release karte hain:
a. Noradrenaline
b. Histamine
c. Acetyl choline
d. GABA

141. HCL ka afraaz hota hai:
a. Parietal cell
b. Chief cell
c. Peptic cell
d. Alveolar cell

142. Neutrophils, Monocytes and Macrophages ke darmiyan kis ka fail mushtarak hai:
a. Immune response
b. Phagocytosis
c. Libration of histamine
d. Destruction of old erythrocytes

143. In angina pectoris which symptom is absent and present in M.I?
a. Chest pain and breathlessness
b. Precipitating factor of exertion and gallop rhythm
c. Breathlessness and gallop rhythm
d. Breathlessness, vomiting, collapse and gallop rhythm

144. Halbeen ki dewarae tashkeel pati hai:
a. 2
b. 3
c. 4
d. None

145. Luaabe duhan kis cheez ke hazma me madad karta hai:
a. Protein and fats
b. Salts and vegetables
c. Sugar and starch
d. None

146. Menstrual blood flow me clotting na hone ki waja hai:
a. Fibrinogen
b. Doderlein bacilli
c. Fibrinolysin
d. Lactobacillus

147. Placenta ki formation hoti hai:
a. After two weeks
b. After three weeks
c. After three months
d. After two months

148. Agar uterine cavity me khoon ka ijtama paya jaye to kahte hai:
a. Hematocolpos

b. Hematometra

c. Pyocolpos

d. All of the above

149. Placenta ka fail hai bataye:

a. Hamal ko barqarar rakhne ke liye hormones enzymes paida karna

b. Hamal ko barqarar rakhne ke liye quwwat bakhshana

c. Hamal ko barqarar rakhne ke liye daurane khoon ko mutwazin rakhna

d. None of the above

150. Palmers sign hamal ke kis zamana me dekha jata hai:

a. Dosre haft eke aakhir me

b. Teesre haft eke

c. 4-8 haft me

d. 6-10 haft me

151. Ek poori muddat hamal ke masheema (Placenta) ka average wiegt kiya hota hai:

a. 500 gm

b. 1000gm

c. 1200 gm

d. 1500 gm

152. Commonest site of ectopic pregnancy:

a. Isthamus

b. Ampulla

c. Infundibulum

d. Abdominal

153. In pneumothorax in which type, valvular air enters the pleural space during inspiration but cannot escape during expiration:

a. Closed

b. Open

c. Tension

d. None of these

154. Hamal ke dauraan Reham aur pistan me numaiya tabdeeli kahlata hai:

a. Hyperplasia

b. Anaplasia

c. Metaplasia

d. None of the above

155. In coma a patient is unconscious but respond tos to strong pain stimulous, he belongs to which grade?

a. Grade 0

b. Grade 1

c. Grade 2

d. Grade 3

156. Waladat ke baad mother ko afraze laban kab ziyadah hota hai:

a. After 3 month

b. After 6 month

c. After 9 month

d. After 12 month

157. Ek aurat ko lactation ke pahle 6 month me kitni zayadh calories darker hoti hai:

a. 300 Kcal/D

b. 400 Kcal/D

c. 550 Kcal/D

d. 800 Kcal/D

158. Bilkhorah kis marz ko kaha jata hai:

a. Daus Salab

b. Salaa

c. Zaufe Shaar

d.Shaare munqalab

159. Dakhas ek marz hai:

a. Hair

b. Nail

c. Jild

d. Old

160. Ufoonat dakhile urooq ho to lahiq hota hai:

a. Humme lazima

b. Humme naiba

c. Humme daira

d. Humme matbaqa

161. Bard wa nafiz malaria me kiyo hota hai?

a. Kurriyate hummara ke totne se

b. Kurriyate hummara ke tadad me kami se

c. Kurriyate hummara ke tauleed me kami se

d. Warme kabid se

162. Warme kabid ka sabab kaun ho sakta hai:

a. Anaemia

b. Nuqs taghzia

c. Nafsuddam

d. Zaheer

163. Malaria me faqaruddam kiyo hota hai:

a. Ghiza mi kami

b. Bukhar ki hiddat wa shiddat

c. Ratoobate jismani ki kami

d. Kurriyate hummarah ki tabahi

164. Bohraan zaiyad ke kitne roaz hai:

a. 8

b. 10

c. 12

d. 14

165. M.I Qalb ke kis hisse me sabse ziyadah hota hai:
a. Left atrium
b. Left ventricle
c. Right atrium
d. Right ventricle

166. Khoon me Australian antigen ki maujoodgi zahir karti hai:
a. Nephritis
b. Cellulitis
c. Hepatitis
d. Warme tihal

167. Parkinsons disease or paralysis agitans most commonly affects the person over the age of:
a. 10 years
b. 30 years
c. 40 years
d. 55 years

168. Shaddle shape nose indicates which disease?
a. AIDS
b. Paralysis
c. Gonorrhoea
d. Syphilis

169. Nabz murtaash ka sabab bataye:
a. Ziyadti hararat
b. Ziyadti ratoobat
c. Ziyadti yabosat
d. Ziyadti barodat

170. Jalinoos bashindah tha:
a. Unan ka
b. Misr ka
c. Roam ka

d. Arab ka

171. Hakeem Ali Geelani kis Oohad KA Tabeeb tha:
a. Oohade Akbari ka
b. Oohade Jhangeer ka
c. Oohade aurangzaibi ka
d. Oohade shah Zufr ka

172. Who is inventor of Polio vaccine?
a. George Sarton
b. Jonas E. Salk
c. John Eghbert
d. George Ibtaheem

173. Hindiustan ka pahla AIDS ka case san me samne aya
a. 1986
b.1979
c. 1981
d. 1085

174. A period of convulsion alternate with unconsciousness without any intervening normal period is called:
a. Grand Mal Epilepsy
b. Tonic Epilepsy
c. Status Epilepsy
d. None of the above

175. Baitul hikmat ke Shobah tarjuma wa talyyaf ka incharge kaun tha:
a. Hanain Ibne Ishaque
b. Yahiya Bar maki
c. Ishaque Ibne Nafis
d. Shabit bin Qarrah

176. Qanooncha kis ki tasneef hai?
a. Alauddin Qarshi
b. Najeebuddin Samarqandi
c. Mohammad bin Chaghmani
d. Ibne Sina

177. Another name of Adult or Juxtaductal coarctatio of aorta is:
a. Preductal
b. Infantile
c. Postductal
d. None of the above

178. Aala Taseed ka name hai:
a. Bhoodar Jantar
b. Doola Jantar
c. Damroo Jantar
d. Pataal Jantar

179. Mugharbal makhsoos hai:
a. Turbud ke liye
b. Soneez ke liye
c. Amla ke liye
d. Ghariqoon ke liye

180. The branch of the science in which deals Origin and growth of the plant is known as:
a. Phytology
b. Phytogeny
c. Phytocrinology
d. None of the above

181. Aqaqia hasil kiya jata hai:
a. Barge Babool
b. Samar babool
c. Chhal babool

d. Gule babool

182. Jo chheezai badan me pahuchti hain wah asar andaz hoti hain:
a. Bil kaifiat, Bil madda, Bil Zohar
b. Bil kaifiat,
c. Bil madda,
d. Sorate nauyia

183. Ek Qeerat hota hai:
a. 4.50 mg
b. 2.50 mg
c. 21 gm
d. 350 mg

184. Polycystic disease of kidney may have cysts in all of the following organs except?
a. Liver
b. Lung
c. Pancreas
d. Spleen

185. Hepatitis B is caused by:
a. DNA Virus
b. RNA Virus
c. Micoplasma
d. Rickettsia

186. Pachak dasti and pachak dashti:
a. Both are same
b. Both terminilogy is wrong
c. Both are terminology of anatomy
d. Both terminologies are different

187. Which Unani drug reduces the cholesterol level?
a. Jozmashal

b. Asaroon

c. Seer

d. Salab mishri

188. Shakar Tighal kis makhaz ki dawa hai:

a. Nabati

b. Haiwani

c. Madani

d. Masnawi

189. Hutchinsons Teeth kis marz ki taraf isharah karta hai:

a. Gonorrhoea

b. AIDS

c. Cancers

d. Congenital syphilis

190. Kis zahar ki sammi alamaat kazaz ki taraf hoti hai:

a. Izaraqi

b. Sankhia

c. Beesh

d. Kutki

191. Typhoid is an infectious disease caused by Salmonella typhi which is a?

a. Gram positive non spore bacteria

b. Gram negative spore bacteria

c. Gram positive spore bacteria

d. Gram negative non spore bacteria

192. Quadriplegia is paralysis of:

a. Upper limb

b. Lower limb

c. Upper and lower limb

d. None of these

193. Urine ka Olive green colour kis zahar khoorani me ho jata hai:
a. Sulphuric acid
b. Carbolic acid
c. Nitric acid
d. Hydrochloric acid

194. Herpes zoster ki muddat hizanat hoti hai:
a. 7-14 days
b. 5-10 days
c. 7-21 days
d. 2-3 days

195. Kala Azar ki muddat hizanat hoti hai:
a. 1-4 days
b. 1-4 months
c. 1-4 years
d. None of the above

196. Sine baloghat ki maloomat ke liye kis qism ki history ki ahamiyat hai:
a. Psycho sexual history
b. Sexual history
c. Family history
d. Endocrinal history

197. After death trachea me Soot ka paya jana dalalat karta hai:
a. Takhneeq
b. Taghreeq
c. Ehraq
d. Taaleeq

198. Dry belly ache kis dhat ki sammi alamat hai:
a. Pb
b. Hg

c. As

d. Sb

199. Generalised convulsion kis zahar khurani me hote hain:

a. Nux vomica

b. Aresenic

c. Mercury

d. Lead

200. Which finger impression is most common?

a. Arch

b. Loops

c. Whirl

d. Composit

MD AMU ENTRANCE EXAMNATION
ANSWER KEY 2004-05

1. A	2. B	3. C	4. C	5. A
6. B	7. C	8. D	9. A	10. B
11. C	12. D	13. A	14. B	15. D
16. D	17. A	18. A	19. C	20. C
21. A	22. D	23. A	24. C	25. D
26. D	27. B	28. B	29. B	30. D
31. B	32. B	33. B	34. A	35. A
36. B	37. D	38. C	39. B	40. B
41. D	42. B	43. A	44. C	45. B
46. B	47. D	48. A	49. B	50. C
51. A	52. A	53. B	54. C	55. B
56. D	57. C	58. B	59. A	60. C
61. A	62. D	63. C	64. A	65. B
66. B	67. D	68. B	69. B	70. C
71. B	72. B	73. C	74. D	75. C
76. D	77. D	78. D	79. D	80. B
81. B	82. B	83. D	84. D	85. C
86. A	87. D	88. A	89. C	90. C
91. C	92. A	93. B	94. C	95. A
96. A	97. C	98. A	99. C	100. A
101. D	102. A	103. A	104. B	105. D
106. B	107. B	108. C	109. C	110. D
111. D	112. D	113. C	114. A	115. A
116. B	117. D	118. C	119. B	120. D
121. D	122. B	123. A	124. D	125. B
126. A	127. B	128. B	129. A	130. B
131. A	132. D	133. B	134. C	135. D
136. D	137. A	138. C	139. B	140. C
141. A	142. B	143. D	144. B	145. C
146. C	147. D	148. B	149. A	150. C
151. A	152. B	153. C	154. A	155. D
156. A	157. C	158. A	159. B	160. A
161. A	162. D	163. D	164. A	165. B

166. C 167. D 168.D 169. A 170. C
171. A 172. B 173. A 174. C 175. A
176. C 177. C 178. C 179. D 180. A
181. A 182. A 183. C 184. B 185. A
186. A 187. C 188 . B189. D 190. A
191. D 192. C 193. B 194. C 195.C
196. D 197. C198. A 199. A 200. B

TEST YOUR KNOWLEDGE (MODEL 1)
(JARAHAT & TST)

1. Nail bed of thumb is supplied by:
a. Radial Nerve
b. Ulnar Nerve
c. Median Nerve
d. None of the above

2. Ludwigs Angina hai:
a. Floor of mouth ka waram
b. Unstable angina
c. Lower oesophagitis
d. None of the above

3. Von Reckhinyhausens disease hai:
a. Generalised neurofibromatosis
b. Plexiform neurofibromatosis
c. Elephentiasis neuromatosis
d. Pachy dermatosis

4. The colour of Oxygen cylinder is:
a. White
b. Black
c. Blue
d. Yellow

5. Chronic smokers me koun sa ulcer common hota hai:
a. Trophic ulcer
b. Tropical ulcer
c. Ischaemic ulcer
d. Bajins ulcer

6. Skin ki premalignant condition koun se hoti hai:

a. Bowens disease

b. Leukoplakia

c. Solar keratosis

d. All of the above

7. Commonest anatomical site of Appendix is:

a. Retrocaecal

b. Pelvicc.

c. Para caecal

d. Subcaecal

8. Amoebic liver abscess sab se common kis hisse me paya jata hai:

a. Lower portion of right lobe

b. Upper portion of right lobe

c. Lower portion of left lobe

d. Upper portion of left lobe

9. Paitt ki chhot me Balancer sign kis uzu ki chhot ki alamat:

a. Spleen

b. Liver

c. Kidney

d. Urinary bladder

10. Coccks Peculiar tumor jism ke kis hissa me paya jata hai:

a. Scalp

b. Neck

c. Chest

d. Abdomen

11. Deep vien thrombosis aam taur par kaha payi jati hai:

a. Calf muscle viens

b. Thigh muscle veins

c. Fore arm deep veins

d. Abdominal veins

12. Dry gangrene is commonest I which disease:
a. Sudden arterial occlusion

b. Slow arterial occlusion

c. Sudden vienus occlusion

d. Diabetic gangrene

13. Rat tail appearance agar Barium shallow kare to kis marz me paya jata hai:
a. Cancer oesophagus

b. Oesophagitis

c. Hiatus hernia

d. Cardiac achalsia

14. Radial nerve ke injured hone ki waja se hota hai:
a. Claw hand

b. Wrist droop

c. Police mans hand

d. None of the above

15. Bacteria for gas gangrene is:
a. Clostridium tatani

b. Strepto cocci

c. Clostridium welchi

d. Staphylococci

16. Halocrine secretion is seen in ………………….. gland:
a. Salivary

b. Mammary

c. Sebaceous

d. Gastric

17. Breast abscess ki sab se ziyadah payi jane wali koun si qism hai?
a. Subareolar abscess
b. Intar mammary abscess
c. Reto mammary abscess
d. Tubercular abscess

18. Meckels Diverticulum kis tarah ke hernia sac me paya jata hai:
a. Littres hernia
b. Mydles hernia
c. Naraths hernia
d. Littles hernia

19. Urine me kis condition me pus cells hone ke sath sterile culture hota hai:
a. Vesical calculus
b. Rena tuberculosis
c. Acute tuberculosis
d. Hydronephrosis

20. The commonest site of carcinoma of tongue is:
a. Tip of the tongue
b. Lateral border
c. Dorsum
d. All of the above

21. Barrets ulcer kiya hota hai:
a. Gastric ulcer
b. Duodenal ulcer
c. Ulcer in lower oesophagus
d. Intestinal ulcer
22. Ano rectal abscess me sab se ziyadah aam qism koun se hai:
a. Perianal

b. Ishiorectal

c. Peelvicrectal

d. Submucous

23. Burn ke mareez me koun sa ulcer hota hai:

a. Trophic ulcer

b. Rodent ulcer

c. Curling ulcer

d. Mouth ulcer

24. Honey bee ke venom ki tadeel ke liye kiya use karna chhaiye:

a. Soda khuradni

b. Sirka

c. Juice of lemon

d. Water

25. Keloid jism ke kis hisse me ziyadah bante hai:

a. Abdomen

b. Pusth par

c. Face par

d. Chest par

26. All have no lymphatics, except:

a. Brain

b. Internal ear

c. Dermis

d. Eye

27. Golf hole ureter is found in:

a. Renal calculus

b. Renal tuberculosis

c. Subarachnoid

d. None of the above

28. Spinal anaesthesia is given in the space of:

a. Epidural space

b. Sub dural space

c. Subarchanoid space

d. None of the above

29. Dermoid tumor is found in:

a. Jild ke kisi bhi hisse me

b. Intestinal wall

c. Abdominal wall

d. Colon

30. Von Reckhiny hausens disease kis tarah ke gene se transmit hoti hai:

a. Autosomal dominant

b. Autosomal recessive

c. Sex linked dominant

d. Sex linked recessive

31. Peela granules nikalta hai:

a. Colocutaneous fistula se

b. Brachial fistula se

c. Actinomycosis se

d. Staphylococal infection se

32. Muscles of tongue supplied by:

a. Linguinal Nerve

b. Glossopharyngeal Nerve

c. Chorda tympani

d. Hypoglossal

33. Cowper's glands open into:
a. Prostatic urethra
b. Membranous urethra
c. Penile urethra
d. Bulbar urethra

34. Hutchisons pupil kis condition me hota hai:
a. Head injury
b. Hemiplegia
c. Tubercular meningitis
d. Syphilis

35. Foramen spinosum se kiya gujarta hai:
a. Maxillary nerve
b. Oclumotor nerve
c. Vertebral artery
d. Middle meningeal artery

36. CVP Line ka complication nahi hai:
a. Pneumothorax
b. Ascites
c. Haemothorax
d. Carotid Artery injury

37. First carpometacarpal joint is a:
a. Hinge joint
b. Saddle joint
c. Elipsoid joint
d. Synovial joint

38. Nipple se bloody discharge hone ki sabab sab se common hai:

a. Duct carcinoma

b. Duct papilloma

c. Fibro adenosis

d. None of the above

39. Carcinoma of stomach kis blood group me common hai:

a. Blood group A

b. Blood group B

c. Blood group AB

d. Blood group O

40. Mandarja zail breast cancer me sab se ziyadah common hai:

a. Lobular carcinoma

b. Ductal carcinoma

c, Inflammatory carcinoma

d. None of the above

41. What is length of normal vasa deference?

a. 30 cm

b. 20 cm

c. 45 cm

d. 60 cm

42. Jaboulays operation kis condition me kiya jata hai:

a. Hernia

b. Undescended testis

c. Retractile testis

d. Hydrocoele

43. HLA- B27 Antigen kin halaat me positive hota hai:

a. AIDS

b. Ankylosing spondilosis

c. Osteomyelitis

d. None of the above

44. Bones me osteoblastic secondaries kis condition me milti hai:

a. Carcinoma breast

b. Carcinoma stomach

c. Carcinoma of prostate

d. All of the above

45. Female Urethra ka narrowest hissa koun sa hota hai:

a. External meatus

b. Membranous urethra

c. Bulbous urethra

d. Internal meatous

46. Thyroid gland ke ander Hot nodule us waqt kahte hain jab:

a. Isotope takeup kam ho

b. Isotope takeup na ho

c. Isotope takeup ziyadah ho

d. None of the above

47. Carcinoma of stomach common hota hai:

a. Cardiac end

b. Greater curvature

c. Lesser curvature

d. Prepyloric region

48. Migrating thrombophelebitis kis cancer ki alamat hai:

a. Ovarian cancer

b. Testicular cancer

c. Breast cancer

d. Gastric cancer

49. Achalasia cardia ke liye koun sa operation kiya jata hai:

a. Gastrectomy

b. Cysto gastrectomy

c. Hellers operation

d. Ramsteds operation

50. Hydatids cyst sab se ziyadah kaha bante hai:

a. Liver

b. Brain

c.Musclea

d. Kidney

51. The nerve supply to pronator teres

a. Median Nerve

b. Radial Nerve

c. Ulnar Nerve

d. Posterior Interosseous Nerve

52. Agar ham Goiter ke mareez me both thyroid lower lobe ko dabaye aur awaaz me stridor paida ho to us ko:

a. Kochers test positive kahte hain

b. Kochers test negative kahte hain

c. Goiter test positive kahte hain

d. Goiter test negative kahte hain

53. The people having small and thick neck me agar Thyroid ka examination karna ho to:

a. Kochers method ka istemaal hota hai

b. Pizzittos method ka istemaal hota hai

c. Razies method ka istemaal hota hai

d. None of the above

54. Haemarroids ke injection lagane me:

a. Gibbons syringe ka istemaal hota hai

b. Hypodermic needle ka istemaal hota hai

c. Gabriels syringe ka istemaal hota hai

d. None of the above

55. Kidney tumor is most common in children is:

a. Neuroblastoma

b. Nephroblastoma

c. Renal cel carcinoma

d. None of the above

56. Brunner's glands are seen in:

a. Jejenum

b. Duodenum

c. Ileum

d. Appendix

57. Buck's fascia is related to:
a. Ischiorectal fascia
b. Thigh
c. Neck
d. Penis

58. Fascia cribosa is related to:
a. Inguinal ring
b. Femoral canal
c. Neck
d. Thigh

59. Ulna ke fracture ke sath agar Radius ka anterior dislocation ho to:
a. Colles fracture kahte hai
b. Galazzis fracture kahte hai
c. Monteggia fracture kahte hai
d. None of the above

60. Subcutaneous tissue ke non suppurative inflammation ko kahte hai:
a. Boil
b. Cellulitis
c. Abscess
d. None of the above

61. Psoas test mojood hotah hai:
a. Pelvic appendicitis
b. Retrocaecal appendicitis

c. Ulcerative colitis

d. Diverticulitis of caecum

62. Sentinal pile isharah karta hai:

a. Ch. Fissure in ano

b. Intestinal tuberculosis

c. Carcinoma of rectum

d. Carcinoma of caecum

63. Ducts of Bellini are found in:

a. Pancreas

b. Submandibular salivary glands

c. Kidney

d. Liver

64. The best treatment of inguinal hernia in children:

a. Herniotomy

b. Herniorrhaphy

c. Hernioplasty

d. None

65. Masana ke cancer me sab se aham khusoosiyat hai:

a. Strangancy

b. Haematuria

c. Refered pain

d. Recuurent infection

66. Murphys sign milta hai:

a. Iltihabe Bancras

b. Iltihabe Mirrara

c. Iltihabe Appendix

d. Iltihabe Colon

67. Huntarian chancre milta hai:

a. Tuberculosis of skin

b. Patient of syphilis

c. Patients of Gonorrhoea

d. None of the above

68. Coldwell-luc operation karte hai

a. Nasal polyp ko nikalne ke liye

a. Cataract ke liye

c. Maxillary sinusitis

d. Gastric ulcer

69. Father of modern surgery is:

a. Joseph lister

b. John hunter

c. Abdul Raisis

d. Buqrat

70. Catgut banta hai:

a. Intestine of cat

b. Intestine of human

c. Intestine of sheep

d. All of the above

71. Filaria ke nateje me testes me jo ratoobat jama hoti hai us ko kahte hai:

a. Chylocele

b. Pyocele

c. Haemocele

d. None of the above

72. Negative occlusion test daleel karta hai:

a. Direct inguinal hernia ki

b. Indirect inguinal hernia ki

c. Hydrocele

d. Obstructive hernia ki

73. Cogh impulses aur Reducibiility alamat hain:

a. Diagnosis of hydrocele

b. Diagnosis of hernia

c. Diagnosis of ectopic ovary

d. Diagnosis of undesceded testis

74. Breast abscess is commonly found in:

a. Lactating mother

b. Unmarried girl

c. mens

d. Mans and womens both

75. Wound suturing me catgut ka istemaal Unani Tabeeb ne kiya :

a. Jlinoos

b. Rhaze

c. Abul Qasim Zohravi

d. None of the above

76. Tashrehi aetibar se Dermoid cyst common hai:

a. tamam jism par

b. At the juncyion of two bones

c. Pusth par

d. Shikam par

77. Sebacoeus cyst aam taur par ziyadah payi jati hai:
a. Tamam jism par
b. Head and glans of penis
c. Head
d. Glans of penis

78. Maqad se khoon ke ikhraj ke sath shaded dard paya jata hai:
a. Bawaseer
b. Nawaseer
c. Inshaqaqe maqad
d. Kharooje maqad

79. Khatna karwana zaroori hota hai:
a. Sartan se mahfooz rahne ke liye
b. Phimosis ki soorat
c. Paraphemosis ki soorat me
d. Both b and c

80. Qarha ziabetus ke indmaal me rukavat paida karte hai:
a. Shakar ki ziyadti
b. Aasab ki
c. Mauf azla ki kamzori
d. All of the above

81. Lock jaw kis disease me hota hai:
a. Rabies
b. Tetanus

c. Meningitis

d. Coma

82.Hydronephrosis hota hai:

a. Unilateral

b. Bilateral

c. Both

d. None of the above

83. Bells palsy kise kahte hai:

a. Radial nerve injury

b. Ulnar nerve injury

c, Facial nerve injury

d. Median nerve injury

84. Ascaris mandarja zail surgical complication paida karte hai:

a. Acute aooendicitis

b. Intestinal obstruction

c. Obstructive Jaundice

d. All of the above

85. Ileostomy:

a. Large intestine ko paitt se bahar nikal kar jorne ko kahte hai

b. Small intestine ko paitt se bahar nikal kar jorne ko kahte hai

c. Stomach ko paitt se bahar nikal kar jorne ko kahte hai

d. None of the above

86. Imperforated anus congenital baccho me hota hai:

a. 3 types

b. 2 types

c. 4 types

d. None of the above

87. Hiatus hernia kise kahte hai:

a. Brain ke herniation ko kahte hai

b. Obstrucying hernia

c. Diaphragmatic hernia

d. Femoral hernia

88. Umblicous hernia ka ilaj ek saal tak ki umr tak yeh hai:

a. Ise waise hi chhor dena chayie

b. Com rakh kar is par bandage lagana chhayie

c. Operation

d. None of the above

89. Projectile vomiting kis me hoti hai:

a. Congenital pyloric stenosis

b. Intestinal obstruction

c. Diverticulosis

d. Appendicitis

90. Cold abscess:

a. Fungal infection se hota hai

b. Tuberculosis me hoti hai

c. Protozoal infection me hoti hai

d. None of the above

91. Inguinal canal ke peche hota hai:

a. Conjoint tendon

b. Fasia transversalis

c. Both a and b

d. None of the above

92. Ek adher umr ki aurat ko solid khane me kam takleef hoti hai banisbat liquid peene me ise kiya marzsakta hai:

a. Cancer oesophagus

b. Reflux oesophagitis

c.Cardia achalasia

d. Stricture oesophagus

93. The common site of cancer of tongue is:

a. Tip

b. Lateral side

c. Dorsum

d. Ventral surface

94. Reactionary haemorrhage occurs at:

a. Upto 24 hours

b. Upto 48 hours

c. In one week

d. Two weeks

95. Which is not complication of duodenal ulcer?

a. Haematemesis

b. Malignancy

c. Stenosis

d. Malena

96. Trendelenberg's sign is a positive in paralysis of all, except?

a. Gluteus medius

b. Gluteus minimus

c. Gluteus maximus

d. Tensor fasia lata

97. Broca's area is concerned with:

a. Word formation

b. Comprehension

c. Repetation

d. Reading

98. Kaboos is seen in :

a. REM sleep

b. Stage II NREM sleep

c. Stage IV NREM sleep

d.Stage I NREM sleep

99. Daily average secretion of Khilt-e-Safra is:

a. 1200 ml

b. 2000 ml

c. 700 ml

d. 225 ml

100. Total volume of C.S.F is:

a. 80 ml

b. 150 ml

c. 600 ml

d. 800 ml

101. Iron and Folic acid supplementation forms:
a. Health promotion
b. Specific promotion
c. Primordial promotion
d. Primary promotion

102. D.P.T vaccine   is given for the prophylaxis of following disease:
a. Ishal, Kali khansi and T.B
b. Diphtheria, Whooping cough and Tetanus
c. Diphtheria, Polio and T.B
d. Ishal galsiwa and tetanus

103. Koplicks spots are seen in the following disease:
a. Rubella
b. Mumps
c. Meascles
d. Chicken pox

104. Shaheeqa kis darja me sab se ziyadah infectious hota hai:
a. In incubation period
b. Catarrhal stage me
c. Proximal stage me
d. Convalscent stage me

105.Which of the following diseae is not come under the surviellance of WHO?
a. Polio
b. Malaria
c. Influenza
d. Varicella

106. Sugar factory me kam karne wale labours me gard wa ghubbar se paida hone wali disease:
a. Byssinosis
b. Bagassosia
c. Farmers lung
d. Pneumoconiosis

107. Deficiency of Phosphorus causes:
a. Osteomalacia
b. Plumbism
c. Khumaq
d. Late coagulation

108. Who discovered O.P.V?
a. Alexender Flaming
b. Sabin
c. Edward jenner
d. Pasteure

109. Peripheral neuritis is caused due to deficiency of:
a. Vitamin C
b. Vitamin D
c. Vitamin B1
d. Vitamin E

110. Which bacteria is responsible for relapsing fever?
a. Ricketsia
b. Borelia
c. Fungus
d. Spirochaetes

111. Horrocks apparatus kis kam ata hai:

a. Bleeching powder ki mikdaar napne ke liye

b. Paani me iodine ki mikdaar napne ke liye

c. Potassium permagnate ki mikdaar napne ke liye

d. Chlorine ki mikdaar napne ke liye

112. Dengue is transmitted by:

a. Anopheles

b. Aedes

c. Bee

d. Culex

113. The term WABA means:

a. Infectious disease

b. Epidemic

c. Endemic

d. Pandemic

114. Kis bemari me badan par chhale nahi nikalte hain:

a. Chicken pox

b. Meascles

c. Polio

d. Rubella

115. Which disease is transmitted from louse?

a. Epidemic typhus

b. Q. fever

c. Oriental sore

d. Scabies

116. Tuberculosis load maloom karne ka sab se good paimana kiya hai:

a. Sputum positive cases

b. Tuberculin positive cases

c. Mortality rate

d. Resistant cases

117. WHO ka head quarter kaha hai?

a. Geneva

b. London

c. Newyork

d. Paris

118. Aangan bari workers kis ki nigraani me kaam karte hai:

a. Wazarate Sehat

b. I .C.D.S Scheem

c. Wazarate taleem

d. WHO

119. Which of the following vaccine is not for typhoid?

a. TAB Vaccine

b. Bivalent anti typhoid vaccine

c. Monovalent anti typhoid vaccine

d. BCG Vaccine

120. Yellow fever is transmitted by :

a. Culex

b. Aedes

c. Anopheles

D. None of the above

121. Cause of Anthrax is:

a. Bacteria

b. Virus

c. Chemical

d. None of the above

122. African sleeping sickness is transmitted by:

a. Sand fly

b. House fly

c. Tse tse fly

d. Bed bug

123. M.T.P Hinduatan me kab lagu hoa?

a. 1972

b. 1971

c. 1975

d. 1980

124. Mental retardation is defined if IQ is below:

a. 90

b. 80

c. 70

d. 60

125. Which of the following causative organism of Malaria is most in the world?

a. P. vivax

b. P. ovale

c. P. falcifarum

d. P. Malaria

126. Cause of Enteric fever is:

a. Solmonella typhi

b. S. para typhi A

c. S. para typhi B

d. All of the above

127. Which of thefollowing disease is not transmitted by mosquitoes?

a. Malaria

b. Filaria

c. Humme Tephodia

d. Dengue

128. Sehat ke ibtadai marakaz (P.H.C) ka aaghaz.......ki report ke baad hoa?

a. Bhuar committee

b. Kartar sing committee

c. Mudaliyar committee

d. None of the above

129. What is daily requirement of protein is?

a. 1 gm/kg body wt

b. 2 gm/kg body wt

c. 3 gm/kg body wt

d. 4 gm/kg body wt

130. Leprosy ki munfaily ka sab se aam sabab hai:

a. Droplets

b. Jild se jild ka taluque

b. Hamile hishiraat

d. none of the above

131. Which of the following is live vaccine?
a. Duck egg vaccine for rabies
b. Salk vaccine
c. TAB Vaccine
d. 17-D yellow fever vaccine

132. Haiza ki waba ko qabon me karne ke liye darje zail me koun sahi hai:
a. Har fard ko teeka lagana
b. Har hafta paani me chlorine milana
c. O.R.S amd Tetracycline ke zariye ilaj karna
d. Notification karna

133. Microfilaria ki janch karne ke liye khoon ka namoona hasil karne ka sahi waqt hai:
a. 08 PM to 10 PM
b. 10 PM to 2 AM
c. 2 AM to 6 AM
d. 08 AM to 10 AM

134. All of the following diseases are seen in India except?
a. Dengue
b. Japanees encephalitis
c. Lassa fever
d. Chicken ghuniya

135.Chemo prophylaxis ki zaroorat aur ahamiyat mandarja zail me kis me nahi hai:
a. Humme Tiphodia
b. Haiza

c. Plague

d. None

136. Which of the following is used as an insecticide?

a. Buzidan

b. Qaranfal

c. Chiraita

d. Darmuna Turki

137. English disease is the term used for:

a. AIDS

b. Chagas disease

c. Chronic bronchitis

d. Rheumatoid arthritis

138. In an epidemic first to be done is:

a. Identify the cases

b. Confirm the diagnosis

c. Identify the prone people

d. Identify the causative factor

139. The risk of bacterial contamination is least with:

a. Ice cream

b. Butter milk

c. Skimmed milk

d. All of those

140. In slaughter house, best to dispose refuses is:

a. Incineration

b. Selling

c. Composting

d. Dumping

141. Which milk is rich of Vitamin K?
a. Human
b. Cow
c. Goat
d. Came

142. Strawberry tongue followed by Respberry tongue is a feature of:
a. Mumps
b. Measles
c. Scarlet
d. Chicken pox

143. Par boiling of paddy helps in retaining:
a. Vitamin A
b. Niacin
c. Vitamin C
d. Thiamine

144. Vitamin C content of seed increases by:
a. Germination
b. Incubation
c. Boiling in warm water
d. Fermentation

145. Alma Ata conference was held in:
a. 1948
b. 1976
c. 1978
d.1965

146. Ragi is a richest source of:

a. Iron

b. Protein

c. Calcium

d. Carbohydrates

147. Sample registration system is done in once in:

a. 6 months

b. 1 year

c. 5 years

d. 10 years

148. Colustrum contains more of ...... than milk:

a. Ca

b. Fe

c. Mg

d. Cu

149. Not a constituent of air:

a. H_2

b. N_2

c. O_2

d. Co_2

150. Wind velocity normally recorded at a height of:

a. 1 mt

b. 10 mts

c. 15 mts

d. 20 mts

151. Who discovered vaccine for Small pox?

a. John Hunter

b. Edward Jenner

c. James Lind

d. Louis Pasteur

152. Negri bodies are found in:

a. Poliomyelitis

b. Viral hepatitis

c. Rabies

d. Encephalitis

153. Another name for German measles:

a. Varicella

b. Rubella

c. Rubeola

d. Pertusis

154. Cholera ke Mareezo me datston ki mahiyat

a. Rice watery

b. Paani ke manind

c. Zaedi mail surkh

d. None of the above

155. Khasra ka teeka kis umr ke bacche me lagaya jata hai:

a. One week

b. 2 Monthh

c. 9 month

d. 12 month

156. Cotton dust ke taluq me rahne se koun sa marz lahique hota hai:

a. Bagassosis

b. Byssinisis

c. Silicosis

d. Anthracosis

157. Marz AIDS me tadreezan koun se cells ka depletion hota hai:

a. T4 cells

b. Beeta cells

c. Yamma cells

d. None

158. Which of the following disease is not arboviral disease?

a. Yellow fever

b. Malaria

c. Japanees encephelatis

d. Bruceelosis

159. WHO ke elaqai daftar kitne mulko me hai?

a. 5

b. 6

c. 7

d. 8

160. Hansens disease ka sabab kiya hai?

a. M. tuberculi

b. M. virus

c. M. leprae

d. None

161. Auditory fatigue occurs at ………….. Hz:

a. 2000

b. 3000

c. 4000

d. 8000

162. Sehat ki policy ke mutalique sabse pahli committee ka naam kiya tha:

a. Mukharjee committee

b. Mudilar committee

c. Buhar committee

d. Chattha committee

163. In India, Rabies free zone is:

a. Goa

b. Lakshwadeep

c. Sikkim

d. Nagaland

164. Aalmi paimane par Yellow fever ke khilaaf koun sa vaccine istemaal kiya jata hai:

a. Ty-21 vaccine

b. 17-D vaccine

c. M-47 vaccine

d. None

165. WHO day kab manaya jata hai?

a. 4th September

b. 6th April

c. Ist December

d. Ist January

166. Which one live vaccine?

a. OPV

b. Hepatitis B

c. TAB

d. Chicken pox

167. Calcium requirement during pregnancy per day is:

a. 2.7 gm

b. 1.6 gm

c. 1.2 gm

d. 3.3 gm

168. In India, death has to registered with in ……….. Days:

a. 5 Days

b. 7 Days

c. 14 Days

d. 11 Days

169. Physical quality of life in India is:

a. 31

b. 43

c. 58

d. 65

170. Hindustan me sab se ziyadah Vitamin C kis se hasil hoti hai:

a. Orange

b. Amla

c. Lemon

D. Imli

171. Chandler's indices is based on:

a. No. of eggs/gm of stool

b. No. of eggs/gm of soil

c. No. of eggs/100gm of stool

d. No. of eggs/100gm of soil

172. Tuberculin test ka result kitni muddat ke baad dekhna hota hai:

a. After 48 hours

b. After 72 hours c.

c. After 96 hours

d. After 24 hours

173. Diq ki tashkhees ka sab se good tareeqa hai:

a. Sputum test

b. X-ray

c. Tuberclin test

d. Patient history

174. The size of Respirable dust is:

a. 1-2 microgram

b. 1-5 microgram

c. 1-10 microgram

d. 1-15 microgram

175. Incubation period of Mumps is:

a. 18 days

b. 16 days

c. 10 days

d. 5 days

176. Poor mans meat is known as:

a. Milk

b. Pulses (Dalein)

c. Fish

d. Eggs

177. In me se kis disease se tahafuz ke liye Oral vaccine de ja sakti hai:

a. Cholera

b. Typhoid

c. Meningococcal meningitis

d. Dengue fever

178. Kis soobah me pellagra aam hai:

a. Kaseeral

b. Andhra

c. UP

d. Delhi

179. When family palnning programme is started?

a. 1947

b. 1950

c. 1952

d. 1960

180. Hind kusht nawaran singh ka taluq kis se hai:

a. Malaria

b. Leprosy

c. Polio

d. Syphilis

181. Population count is taken on:

a. 1st January

b. 1st March

c. 1st July

d. 1st Aug

182. Bysinossis is common in:

a. Weavers

b. Spinners

c. Growers

d. Dyers

183. Upper limit of tolerance of noice/day is:

a. 10 dB

b. 85 dB

c. 90 dB

d. 160 dB

184. Pregnant lady ko aam taur se kitni extra calories leena chhaiye:

a. 100 calories

b. 300 calories

c. 500 calories

d. 700 calories

185 Which of the following foodborne disease is fingal origin?

a.. Lathyrism

b. Endemic asites

c. Botulism

d. Aflatoxin

186. Neonatal period birth se start hota hai aur birth se kitne days tak rahta hai:

a. 7 days

b. 14 days

c. 21 days

d. 28 days

187. Children ki birth se kitne arsa baad aam taur se mothers ko apne bacchon ko doodh pilana chhaiye:

a. Fauran

b. After 3 days

c. After one week

d. After two weeks

188. In India which is most common cause of blindness:

a. Trachoma

b. VitaminA deficiency

c. Glaucoma

d. Cataract

189. Mammography is used in diagnosis of which disease?

a. Cancer cervix

b. Cancer breast

c. Oral cancer

d. Lung cancer

190. What is daily requirement of salt in Hypertensive patient?

a. 4-6 gm

b. 8-10 gm

c. 12-14 gm

d. 16-18 gm

191. Which of the following blood lipid is beneficial for health?

a. Total cholesterol

b. LDL cholestrol

c. HDL Cholestrol

d. Triglycerides

192. Western blot test is used in the diagnosis of:

a. Rabies

b. Poliomyelitis

c. Tetanus

d. AIDS

193. Fernandez reaction kis test me paya jata hai?

a. Lepromin test

b. Montoux test

c. Shick test

d. None of the above

194. Lock jaw kis disease me paya jata hai?

a. Whooping cough

b. Tuberculosis

c. Tetanus

d. Typhoid fever

195. Trichiasis kis disease ki khusoosiat hai:

a. Cataract

b. Trachoma

c. Glaucoma

d. Vitamin A deficiency

196. Black water fever is a complication of:

a. P. Vivax

b. P. Ovale

c. P.Malariae

d. P. Falciparum

197. Rabies me zakham ki safai ke liye mandarja zial me se kise istemaal nahi karna chhaiye:

a. Soap

b. Alcohol

c. Iodine

d. Carbolic acid

198. Ancyclostoma duodenale se koun se disease hoti hai:

a. Ascariasis

b. Hookworm infection

c. Dracunculiasis

d. Leptospirosis

199. Diethyl carbamazine citrate kis disease me use karte hai?

a. Yellow fever

b. Guinea worm disease

c. Lymphatic filariasis

d. Leptospirosis

200. ORS me potassium chloride kitne gram hota hai?

a. 3.5 gm

b. 2.5 gm

c. 1.5 gm

d. 0.5 gm

TEST YOUR KNOWLEDGE (MODEL 1)
ANSWER KEY(JARAHAT & TST)

1. A	2. A	3. A	4. B	5. C
6. D	7. A	8. B	9. A	10. A
11. A	12. D	13. D	14. B	15. C
16. C	17. B	18. A	19. B	20. B
21. C	22. A	23. C	24. A	25. B
26. A	27. B	28. C	29. C	30. A
31. C	32. D	33. C	34. A	35. D
36. A	37. B	38. B	39. A	40. B
41. C	42. D	43. B	44. C	45. A
46. C	47. D	48. D	49. C	50. A
51. A	52. A	53. B	54. C	55. B
56. B	57. D	58. B	59. C	60. B
61. B	62. A	63. C	64. A	65. B
66. B	67. B	68. A	69. A	70. C
71. A	72. A	73. B	74. A	75. C
76. B	77. B	78. C	79. D	80. D
81. B	82. C	83. C	84. D	85. B
86. B	87. C	88. AB	89. B	90. B
91. C	92. C	93. B	94. A	95. A
96. C	97. A	98. A	99. C	100. B
101.B	102.B	103.C	104.B	105.B
106.B	107.A	108.B	109.C	110.A
111.D	112.B	113.B	114.C	115.A
116.A	117.A	118.B	119.D	120.A
121.A	122.C	123.B	124.C	125.A
126.D	127.B	128.A	129.A	130.B
131.D	132.B	133.B	134.C	135.A
136.A	137.C	138.B	139.B	140.A
141.B	142.C	143.D	144.A	145.C
146.C	147.B	148.C	149.A	150.B
151.B	152.C	153.B	154.A	155.C
156.B	157.A	158.B	159.B	160.C

161.C 162.C 163.A 164.B 165.B
166.A 167.C 168.B 169.B 170.B
171.B 172.B 173.A 174.B 175.A
176.B 177.B 178.B 179.C 180.B
181.C 182.B 183.B   184.B 185.D
186.D 187.A 188 .D 189.B 190.A
191.C 192.D 193.A 194.C 195B
196.D   197.C 198.B 199.C 200.B

TEST YOUR KNOWLEDGE (MODEL 2)
(Amraz-e-Niswan and Moalajat)

1. P^H of vagina during reproductive period:
a. 3
b. 5.5
c. 4.5
d. 7

2. Pre-cocious menarche kahte hai:
a. 8 Years ki umr me haiz ka aana
b. Before 10 Years ki umr me haiz ka aana
c. Before 15 Years ki umr me haiz ka aana
d. After 15 Years ki umr me haiz ka aana

3. Surkh baddah furj ka sabab hai:
a. Streptococcous
b. Staphylococcus
c. Gonococcus
d. All of the above

4. DUB ka sabab ho sakta hai:
a. Amraze Reham
b. Zaufe Reham
c. Amraze Dam
d. Both b and c

5. Azlate Reham ki dabajat kitni hoti hai:
a. 8 to 10 mm
b. 10 to 12 mm
c. 6 to 8 mm
d. 4 to 6 mm

6. Human milk ke 100 ml me kitni calories hoti hai
a. 60

b. 75

c. 55

d. 57

7. During reproductive period in which organs Tuberculosis is most common in?

a. Ghisai unqurreham

b. Cervix

c. Fallopian tube

d. Ovaries

8. Endometriosis ki alamat hai:

a. Tamshi khoon ka ruk jana

b. Tamshi khoon ka ziyadah ho jana

c. Tamshi khoon ka kam ho jana

d. None of the above

9. The tibbi term for 'Inversion of Uterus' is:

a. Zalaq ul Reham

b. Nutu ur Reham

c. Irtikas ur Reham

d. All of the above

10. The term Zujajak means:

a. Ampula

b. Fornix

c. Fourchette

d. Isthmus

11. Monozygotic twins ki incidence hasbe zail hai:

a. 1:100

b. 1:200

c. 1: 150

d. 1: 250

12. The commonest cause of cancer of cervix:
a. Adeno carcinoma
b. Transitional cell carcinoma
c. Squamous cell carcinoma
d. Secondaries

13. Wah ghair tabai Aana jis me One alae of sacrum ka development nahi hota hai:
a. Rober pelvis
b. Naegles pelvis
c. Android pelvis
d. Gynaeecoid pelvis

14. Neonate ka Apgar score agar 0.3 ho to kis qism me shumaar kiya jata hai:
a. Pallida
b. Livida
c. Moderate
d. Good

15. Rectal examination kab kiya jata hai:
a. Ovaries ko aasni se mahsoos karne ke liye
b. Jab vaginal examination assan na ho
c. Utero sacral ligament mahsoos karne ke liye
d. All of the above

16. Conjoint twins aam taur par hote hain:
a. Binovutes
b. Uniovutes
c. Trisomy
d. None of the above

17.What is iron binding capacity during pregnancy?
a. 305+32 microgm/100/ml
b. 300+20 microgm/100/ml
c. 250+30 microgm/100/ml

d. 350+30 microgm/100/ml

18. Alqanoon fit Tibb ke kis jild me amraze niswan ka tazkirah hai:
a. Volume I
b. Volume II
c. Volume III
d. Volume IV

19. Hikkatul furj ke sath mahbali akharajat ki ziyadti ka sabab hota hai:
a. Trichmoniasis
b. Candida
c. Gonococci
d. Chalmydia

20. The size of the Uterus is :
a. 3.5 cm
b. 7.5 x 5 x 2.5 cm
c. 3.5 x 2.5 x 1.8 cm
d. 10 cm

21. The number of layers in Reham are:
a. Two
b. Three
c. Four
d. Only one

22. Vesicular mole Hamal ke kis hafte se banna shuru hota hai:
a. In first 4 weeks
b. In first 8 weeks
c. In first 2 weeks

d. In first 12 weeks

23. Istaqrare hamal agar Qazfain me ho to kis hissa me hota hai:

a. Barzakh

b. Farakhta

c. Qumaa

d. Khulai hissa

24. Kitabul Mansoori fit Tibb ke musanif koun hai?

a. Buqrat

b. Ibne sina

c. Zakaria Rhazes

d. Ali bin abbas majoosi

25. Chha hafte me bacche ki lambai c.m kitni hoti hai?

a. 0.5 cm

b. 1 cm

c. 1.5 cm

d. 2 cm

26. Mandarja zail Kitabo me se Buqrat kis kitab ke musanif nahi hai:

a. Kitabul ajanaa

b. Kitabul aujaaunnisa

c. Kitabul junaian

d. Kitabul maulood

27. Auratto me testosterone ki miqdaar kitni hpti hai:

a. 0.1 to 0.5

b. 1 to 2

c. 0.2 to 0.4

d. None of the above

28. Which of the following glands have no glands?

a. Cervix

b. Endometric

c. Vulva

d. Vagina

29. Turners syndrome me chromosomes ki tadaad:

a. 47 XXY

b. 46 XY

c. 45 XO

d. 44 XX

30. Mandarja zail amraz me se ehtabas tams paya jata hai:

a. Turners syndrome

b. Sheehans syndrome

c. Frothlics syndrome

d. All of the above

31. Jism Asfar are seen in:

a. Cortex

b. Medulla

c. Fallopian Tubes

d. Uterus

32. Placenta ke kharij ho jane ke baad haemostatic ka sabse aham sabab kiya hai:

a. Uterine contraction

b. Uterine retraction

c. Thrombosis

d. Myotemporade

33. Uterine inertia, labour ki kis stage me complicationpaida karta hai

a. I stage

b. II stage

c. III stage

d. All of the above

34. Koun sa ligament Reham ke kharoojulreham ke liye sab se ziyadah zimedar hota hai:

a. Round ligament

b. Broad ligament

c. Cardinal ligament

d. Vaginal fascia

35. During Puberty in which stage the breast development occurs:

a. Pre puberty Stage

b. 1st stage of puberty

c. 2nd stage of puberty

d. 3rd stage of puberty

36. Face presentation ka denominator kiya hai:

a. Nose

b. Mentum

c. Lips

d. Anus

37. Nasoor e Reham:

a. Ek marzi kaifiat hai

b. Qaroohe Reham

c. Akla Reham ke complication me hai

d. Sartane Reham

38. Vaginal fistula ke aqsaam hai:

a. Vesico vaginal

b. Recto vaginal

c. Urethro vaginal

d. All of the above

39. Shaqaqurreham ki soorat me lahique hota hai:

a. Shadeed dardaza

b. Reham ki sakht yaboosat

c. Usre waladat

d. All of the above

40. Tuwarad is a sign of:

a. Menarche

b. Menopause

c. Puberty

d. Climacterium

41. Hikkaturreham ki kitni iqsam hain:

a. 2

b. 5

c. 3

d. 4

42. Criteria of normal pregnancy me koun se baat shamil nahi hai:

a. Delivery between 38-42 weeks

b. Foetal weight 2.5 kg

c. Less maternal complication

d. Single baby

43. Haad Iltihab Reham ke asbab hain:

a. Naffasi infection

b. Abortive infection

c. Salpingitis

d. All of the above

44. The term Istihaza is:

a. Menorrhagia

b. Metrorrhagia

c. Polymenorrhoea

d. DUB

45. In developed country the cause of PID:

a. Gonprrhoea

b. IUCD

c. Abortion

d. Chlamydia infection

46. Klinefelters syndrome me chrompsome ki Tadad kiya hoti hai:

a. 45 XO

b. 46 XY

c. 47 XXY

d. 44 XX

47. Candida albicans se koun se disease hoti hai?

a. Amoebic vaginitis

b. Giardiasis

c. Ulcers

d. None of the above

48. Blood supply of uterus is:

a. Uterine artery

b. Ovarian artery

c. Vaginal artery

d. All of the above

49. Chorio carcinoma kis ka malignant tumor hota hai:

a. Chorionic Trophoblast

b. Chorionic Cyto Trophoblast

c. Chorionic mole

d. None of the above

50. Prolonged mensus without affecting the duration and amount of flow is seen in:

a. Qillat Tams

b. Ta'ddid Tams

c. Tahat Tams

d. Kasrat Tams

51. Alhavi me amraze niswan ka tazkirah kis volume me hai:

a. 7th volume

b. 9th volume

c. 6th volume

d. 8th volume

52. Ilmul Qabalat ka tazkirah kis Pappyrus me hai:

a. Barlan Pappyrus

b. Kahoon Pappyrus

c. Abrus Pappyrus

d. All of the above

53. Junain ki iswate qalb sab se pahle kis ne daryaft kiya:

a. Buqrat

b. Herophilus

c. Jalinoos

d. All

54. Ceaserian section ke zariyah waladat ka tafsili zikr aur tareeqa kis kitab me maujood hai:

a. Alhavi

b. Alqanoon

c. Kitabul jarahat

d. Sashrath Samhatta

55. McIndole's and Williiam's surgery are the choice in:

a. Inqilab ur Raham

b. Bawasir Reham

c. Inshiqaq ur Reham

d. Rataq

56. Chocholate Cysts of the Ovary is a sign of:

a. Usr Tams Sanawi

b. Tahat Tams

c. Ta'ddud Tams

d. Kasrat Tams

57. Warme Jasiah kis ko kahte hai:

a. Reham ki rasooli

b. Qarooh zakhm Reham

c. Mehabal ka waram

d. Reham ka sartani sakht waram

58. Istarkha fame Reham ki makhsoos dawa hai:

a. Aqaqia

b. Shib

c. Juffat baloot

d. All of the above

59. Janain me erythropoiesis hamal ke kis hafte me hoti hai:

a. 6

b. 4

c. 2

d. 10

60. Jin drugs se junain ki hifazat hoti hai:

a. Advia muqawwi

b. Advia qalbia

c. Mudir Advia

d. All of the above

61. Ehtabase Tams ka sabab nahi hai:

a. Qilate khoon

b. Ghilzate khoon

c. Kasrate istifragh

d. Riqate khoon

62. Ikhtanaqur-reham me nabz wa tanafus:

a. Hararate gharizi ghat jati hai

b. Hararate gharizi increase ho jati hai

c. Hararate gharizi mutasir nahi hoti hai

d. Reham me ghilzat ho jati hai

63. Nafakhe reham ka sabab hai:

a. Sue mizaj har

b. Sue mizaj yabis

c. Zaufe Reham

d. Sue mizaj barid

64. Bawaseer e Reham me koun se khilt sabab hoti hai:

a. Dam

b. Dam wa Safra

c. Sauda

d. Balgham khaam

65. Farbhai me uqr ka khaas sabab:

a. Kasrate ratoobat

b. Kasrate baroodat

c. Fame Reham me shameen ka jama hona

d. Reham ka farba hona

66. Mudir laban ka ilaj hasbe zail usool par karte hai:

a. Mudir Tams

b. Mudir Boul

c. Habis Tams

d. Muqawwiyat

67. Kasrate laban ki soorat me koun si dawa mufeed hai:

a. Mazo

b. Samag arabi

c. Tukhm Kasoos

d. Tukhm Hulba

68. Waladat ke baad neonate ki jild:

a. Raqeeq aur sard hoti hai

b. Raqeeq aur khusk hoti hai

c. Raqeeq aur garam hoti hai

d. None

69. Paidaish ke baad amale Razaat kab munasib hai:

a. Jab doodh ki rangat badal jati hai

b. Jab doodh motadil ho jay

c. Jab mareeza sehat mand ho jaye

d. None

70. Ehtabase Tams ki soorat me boul ka rang:

a. Siyahi mail

b. Zardi mail

c. Sufaidi mail

d. None

71. Alhavi ki koun si jild me Ilmul Qabalat ka bayaan hai:

a. 6

b. 7

c. 8

d. 9

72. Injection toxoid un tamam aurton ko diya jata hai:

a. Hamla me

b. After delivery

c. After one week of delivery

d. After ten days of delivery

73. B.C.G and OPV Un tamam childrens ko diya jata hai:

a. Jo house me paida ho

b. Jo hospital me paida ho

c. In both condition

d. None of the above

74. Hindustan me taqreeban har saal kitne bachhe paida hote hai:

a. 5 cror

b. two cror fifty thousands

c. One cror fifty lac

d. Six cror

75. 100 ml mother ke milk me taqreeban kitni fat hoti hai:

a. 5 gm

b. 2 gm

c. 3.5 gm

d. 14 gm

76. Neonate me hypothermia ki taareef ye hai

a. Less than 35.5 C^0

b. More than 36.0 C^0

c. 345 C^0

d. 37 C^0

77. Which of the following is the most painful condition in Muzmin Iltihab Farj?

a. Leukoplakia

b. Tuberculous Vulvitis

c. Actinomycosis

d. Vulvul Warts

78. Bartholins glands are open in:

a. Inner surface of Labium minus

b . Outer surface of Labium minus

c. Inner surface of Labium major

d. Outer surface of Labium major

79. 100 ml mother ke doodh me kitni calories hoti hai:

a. 60

b. 80

c. 67

d. 72

80. In which stage of Qarooh Farj Aathiski, Salil are found?

a. Ulcerative Condylamata

b. Granuloma Inguinale

c. Chancroid Ulcers

d. Gummatous Ulcers

81. What is not an event of Behcet's syndrome?

a. Recurrent oral ulceration

b. Recurrent genital ulceration

c. Iridocyclitis

d. Elephantiasis of Clitoris

82. The normal length of Bazar is:

a. 0.5 cm

b. 1 cm

c. 1.5 cm

d. 2.5 cm

83. Ph of Mehbal in Child bearing stage is:

a. 5.7

b. 4

c. 7

d. 4.5

84. Aash Jau ki pichkari kis me mufeed hai:

a. Iltihab Mehbal

b. Hikkatul Farj

c. Surkhbadi Iltihab Farj

d. Azm ul bazaar

85. Amber coloured watery discharge is sign of:

a. Ca. Fallopian Tube

b. Salpingitis

c. Parametritis

d. Para ovarin cyst

86. Vaginisomus means:

a. Tazeeq Mehbal

b. Istirkha Mehbal

c. Tashanuj Mehbal

d. A & C

87. Wajaur Raham bil sabab Sue Mizaj Har me:

a. Kasrat Haiz hota hai

b. Haiz sufaidi mayal surkh hota hai

c. Haiz Ghaleez aur surkh siyahi hota hai

d. All of the above

88. Marham Dakhalyoon is used as a Hamool in:
a. Bawasir Reham

b. Sailanur Raham

c. Sartan ur Reham

d. Takul Unaq

89. Grape shaped polyp is seen in:
a. Mucous Polyp

b. Fibroid Polyp

c. Placental Polyp

d. Sarcoma Polyp

90. Most common cause of Muzmin Waram Reham is:
a. Gonorrhea

b. Syphilis

c. Tuberculosis

d. All

91. Most common cause of Mailan Reham Khalfi Harki is:
a. Congenital

b. Puerperal

c. Nulliparous

d. PID

92. The types of Tanasuli Saqoot are:
a. 2

b. 3

c. 4

d. 5

93. Laxity of Pouch of Douglas is called:

a. Cystocele

b. Enterocele

c. Rectocele

d. Urethrocele

94. Inqilabur Reham is common in which trimester of pregnancy:

a. First

b. Second

c. Third

d. None

95. A Cup like depression of the abdomen is a feature of:

a. Sula Reham leefi

b. Isthirqa Mehbal

c. Mailanur Reham

d. Munqalibur Reham

96. How many types of Sulat ur Reham are present:

a. 2

b. 3

c. 6

d. 5

97. Adeemul Hamal women are more prone to:

a. Uterine Prolapse

b. Uterine Sarcoma

c. Uterine Fibroids

d. Uterine Polyp

98. Most common abortions seen in between 80-90 days are caused by:

a. Ghalba Hararat

b. Ghalba Barudat

c. Ghalba Ratubat

d.Ghalba Yabusat

99. What is not suggested in Sue Ratubat Reham?

a. Arq Baid Musk

b. Arq Baranjasif

c. Majun Falasifa

d. Maul Leham

100. The term 'Rahmi Ijtima Ghaza' is referred to:

a. Hydrometra

b. Pyometra

c. Physiometra

d. None

101. Khibta name hai:

a. Suda barid kharji ka

b. Suda har kharji ka

c. Suda shirki ka

d. Shaqeeqa ka

102. Haqeeqi Asaba kise kagte hai:

a. Dard ke sath azlati tasanuj na ho

b. Dard ke sath azlati tasanuj ho

c. Dard ke sath tasanuj ka paya jana zaroori hai

d. None of the above

103. Azamul ras haqeeqi me amooman hota hai:

a. Darooz alaihida ho jati hai

b. Vareed ubhri hoi milti hai

c. Sar ka agla hissa barh jata hai

d. Sar ka pichla hissa ziyzdah barh jata hai

104. Warme aghshia dimagh batadreez:

a. Gardan ke azlaat dhele ho jate hai

b. Gardan ke azlaat rigid ho jate hai

c. Pust ke azlaat istarkha ho jate hai

d. None of the above

105. Fasade fikr kahte hain:

a. Mareez kisi baat ko bilkul sooch na sake

b. Soochta to hai magar bhool jata hai

c. Kuch yaad rakhta hai kuch bhool jata hai

d. Soochta kam hai lekin bhoolta bilkul nahi hai

106. Laqwa tasanuji me marz shuru hone ke kitne dinon ke baad mushily deena hota hai:

a. 21 Days

b. 14 days

c. 4-7 days

d. Hasbe zaroorat in me se kisi bhi din

107. Kasham kis uzu ka marz hai:

a. Ear

b. Nose

c. Eye

d.Tongue

108. Dawi (Tinitus) se muraad hai:

a. Bahrapan

b. Farzi aur khayali awazain jin ka vajood kharij me nahi hota hai magar insaan in ko suntan hai

c. Neend ki bimaari

d. Waham

109. Bauwattain kis uzu ka marz hai:

a. Kidney

b. Masana

c. Anaf

d. Chashm

110. Acute M.I ke fauran baad Aspirin ki pahli khurak kitni hoti hai:

a. 500 mg

b. 1000 mg

c. 150 mg

d. 300 mg

111. Haemic murmur kin halaat me sunai parta hai?

a. Khoon ki kami me

b. Valular heart diseases me

c. Disease of lungs

d. Disease of aorta

112. Malignant hyprtension ki tashkhees ki jati hai:

a. Raised B.P

b. convulsion

c. Papilloedema

d. Haematuria

113. Bohare qalbi me ho sakta hai except?

a. Tanafus azim ho lekin nabz saghir

b. Tanafus azim ho lekin nabz taweel

c. Nabz aur Tanafus dono saghir ho

d. Nabz aurTanafus dono azim ho

114. Maut ke waqt ki nabz?

a. Sulb wa bate

b. Layyan wa bate

c. Taweel wa Duwi

d. Zaeef wa zulfitra

115. Localized wheezing bilumoom sunai deti hai:

a. Lobar pneumonia me

b. Riya jis me jisme gharib ka hona

c. Bronchiectasis

d. Kharaje riya

116. Diq me riya ke alawah umoomi taur par koun si sakht mutasir hoti hai?

a. Pericardium

b. Peritoneum

c. Spine

d. Testes

117. Lobular pneumonia me waram paya jata hai:

a. Ek janib ke riya me

b. Ek janib ke riya k eek hissa me

c. Ek janib ke riya ke mutaddid hisson me

d. Dono janib ke riya me

118. Maroof marz waham ka madda meda me kis jagah maujood hota hai?

a. Meda ko aster karne wali bairooni jhilli

b. Fame meda me

c. Jarme meda me

d. Khumle meda

119. Madatul batan se kiya muraad hai:

a. Darde shikam

b. Sue hazam

c. Ishal

d. Zaufe jigar

120. Sarkhas kis deedan ki makhsoos dawa hai:

a. Dedane tuaa

b. Dedane sighar

c. Hubbul qaraa

d. All of the above

122. The Mutradif of Jamrah is:

a. Jamrah Khabisa

b. Qurooh Balkhiya

c. Shabe Chiragh

d. All

123. The Mutradif of Qarha Rakhwa is:

a. Atishak Moarasi

b. Aatisak Iktasabi

c. Aatishak Majazi

d. None

124. What is the Mutradif of Khayarjal?
a. Jhangasa
b. Warm Maghabin
c. Warm Kunjaran
d. All

125. Amraze jigar me Sibr ka istemaal:
a. Be khatar karna chhaiye
b. Bilkul nahi karna chhaiye
c. Islaah ke baad hi karna chhaiye
d. Hajat shaded ho to islaah ke baghair hi kar lena chhaiye

126. Plain X ray abdomen me under the diaphragm se confirmative diagnosis hoti hai:
a. Istisqai Tabli ki
b. Perforated peptic ulcer ki
c. Ascites ki
d. Intestinal obstrucyion ki

127. Zaufe Tihal ki kis qism me sankhia aur us ke murakkabat ka istemaal mufeed hai:
a. Waram
b. Leukaemia
c. Both
d. None

128. Hazale kuliya ka sabab ho sakta hai:
a. Jamaa ki kasrat
b. Advia mushila ka bafrat istemaal
c, Advia mudiraat ka bafrat istemaal

d. All of the above

129. I like open air is the:
a. Particular symptoms
b. Common symptoms
c. General symptoms
d. Characteristic symptoms

130. Boul ke rozana akhraj me kis qadr kami waqai ho jai to us ko oligouria kahte hai:
a. 700 ml
b. 600 ml
c. 500 ml
d. 500 ml se kam

131. Boule ashqar nishandahi karta hai:
a. Humme diq ki
b. Humme lisqa ki
c. Humme medi ki
d. Sarsam har ki

132. Sweat ki kasrat, ikhtalaj aur Rasha kis uzu ki marzi alamat hai:
a. Qalb
b. Dimagh
c. Thyroid gland ki
d. Pituitary gland

133. Kis beemari me pre Tibial myxoedema paya jata hai:
a. Hyperthyroidism

b. Myxoedema

c. Heart failure

d. Both a and c

134. Thyroxin ki kami ki soorat me jo mallomat milti hain wah baru had tak:

a. Ghalba balgham ki alamat se

b. Ghalba dam ki alamat se

c. Ghalba sauda ki alamat se

d. Ghalba safra ki alamat se

135. Joshandah haleela ke zariye:

a. Balgham ko nuzaj dete hai

b. Safra ko kharij karte hai

c. Akhlate ghaliz ko raqeeq karte hai

d. Neend late hai

136. Jawarish Jalinoos kis umr me ziyadah munasib hai:

a. Sine Tifoliya

b. Sine Baloghat

c. Sine Shaikhokhat

d. Sine Kaholat

137. Aaqoona ki shikayat aam hai

a. In males

b. In females

c. Both

d. None of the above

138. Jamaa wa jalaq zaufe baah ka sabab ho to ibtida me kis tarah ki dawa di jaygi:

a. Muqawwi wa muharik

b. Musakin wa mubarid

c. Munawim wa mukhadir

d. Munaash wa muharik

139. Sozaki maddah ke khoon me shareek hone se paida hota hai:

a. Pyaemia

b. Anaemia

c. Haemorrhage

d. Haematuria

140. Nawaseer kahte hai:

a. Maqad ke gahre zakhm ko

b. Maqad ke satahi zakhm ko

c. Maqad ke shaded waram ko

d. Maqad ke khafeef waram ko

141. Busoore ghariba ki qismai hain kul:

a. 2

b. 4

c. 5

d. 6

142. Juzame khudri me payi jati hai:

a. Gantth khudir ke sath

b. Gantth mamooli khudir ke sath

c. Khudir Gantth ke baghair

d. All of the above

143. Dabeela ki shakal hoti hai:
a. Goul nookdar
b. Nookdar
c. Goul aur be nookdar
d. Chapta aur khurdara

144. Aag se jal jane par bartna jahiye:
a.Marham Raal
b. Marham Sufaida
c. Marham Naura
d. None of the above

145. Acute Malaria me hamla auraton me chloroquin de ja sakti hai ki nahi:
a. Yes
b. No
c. Never
d. Some times

146. Dengue fever kis virus se hota hai:
a. Flavi virus
b. Retro virus
c. Toga virus
d. Astro virus

147. Ghib Muzaif kahte hain ud bukhar ko jis me:
a. Rozana ek shaded bari aati hai
b . Rozana two shaded bari aati hai
c. Rozana ek khafeef bari aati hai
d. Rozana ek din me three or four bariya aati hai

148. What type of Warm is Saqeerus?
a. Warm Aakla
b. Warm Barid
c. Warm Sulb
d. All

149. Shatrul Ghib paida hota hai
a. Balgham and Dam se
b. Balgham and Sauda se
c. Balgham only
d. Balgham and Safara se

150. The diagnosis of typhoid fever in first week through:
a. Blood culture
b. Widal test
c. Stool culture
d. Urine culture

151. Talayyanud dimagh me koun se Talayyan hoti hai:
a. Talayyan abaiyaz
b. Talayyan ahmar
c. Talayyan asfar
d. All of the above

152. Warme uslul uzn kis ghudah ka waram hai:
a. Warme ghudah darqiah
b. Warme ghudah nakfia
c. Warme ghudah tahtul lisaan
d. Warme ghudah luabia

153. Saraa me kiya hota hai:
a. Hont phat jate hain
b. Gums se bleeding hoti hai
c. Toungue kat jati hai

d. Epistaxsis hoti hai

154. Hizyan is the vital sign of:
a. Ghib Khalisa
b. Ghib Ghair Khalisa
c. Ghib Maftara
d. Ghib Muharriqa

155. Nafsuddam sabab ha qalbi amraz ka:
a. Mitral stenosis
b. Mitral regurgitation
c. VSD
d. Aortic stenosis

156. Salaa kis halat ko kahte haii:
a. Hairs ka safaid hona
b. Chandiya saaf hoona
c. Hairs jharna
d. Kasafate shaar

157. Uqab kis marz ko kahte hai:
a. Falik itrafi ko
b. Istarkah ko
c. Laqwa ko
d. Kazaz ko

158. Balahat dar asal wah marzi alamat hai jis me:
a. Insaan me aqal kam hoa karti hai
b. Insaan me aqal tabai hoa karti hai
c. Insaan me aqal me kharabi hoa karti hai
d. Insaan me aqal bilkul nahi payi jati hai

159. Nabz mukhtalif (Pulsus alternans) payi jati hai:

a. Aortic stenosis

b. Endocarditis

c. Pan cystolic murmur

d. H.O.C.M

160. Dawai bahrozah kis marz me istemaal karte hai:

a. Nephritis

b. Gonorrhoea

c. Syphilis

d. Urinary bladder ulcer

161. Kis marz me negri bodies payi jati hai:

a. Hepatitis B

b. HIV

c. Rabies

d. Varicella

162. Anxiety paida hoti hai:

a. Ghalba dam se

b. Ghalba safra se

c. Ghalba balgham se

d. Ghalba sauda se

163. Bahtul soot kahte hai:

a. Jis me awaaz band ho jati hai

b. Jis me awaaz moti ho jati hai

c. Jis me awaaz bareek ho jati hai

d. Jis me awaaz tez ho jati hai

164.Zakhm ko mail aur peep waghairah se is qadar saaf karta hai ki is ke muqable me koi doosri dawa nahi hai:

a. Maaul buzoor

b. Maaul usal

c. Maaul jubn

d. Maaul shaeer

165. Qaroohe saaiya ki bairooni satah kaisi hoti hai:

a. Mamooli khurdari

b. Bahut khurdari

c. Chikni

d. Kharash dar

166. Bawaseer Rehami ka muqaame marz hota hai:

a. Whole uterus

b. Cervix

c. Fame Reham

d. b and c

167. Boule kurrasi ek qism hai:

a. Boule sabz

b. Boule asafar

c. Boule ahmar

d. Boule aswad

168. Hajabe Hazij ke tasanuj ka natijah hota hai:

a. Jishaa

b. Fawaq

c. Wajaul fawad

d. Nafkha

169. Sarra me tasanujka sabab hota hai:

a. Roohe nafsaani ke raston ka mukkamal sudda

b. Dimaghi shiryaan ka mikkamal sudda

c. Roohe nafsaani ke raston ka na mukkamal sudda

d. Dimaghi shiryaan ka na mikkamal sudda

170. Nabz Minshari is found in:

a. Pneumonia

b. Hypertension

c. Pleural effusion

d. Pleurisy

171. Marz Zaghoth me:

a. Dimagh bheej jata hai

b. Imtila ho jata hai

c. Iltihab ho jata hai

d. Sudda paida ho jata hai

172. Khasam aisa marz hai jis me:

a. Hisse zaiqa madoom ho jati hai

b. Hisse shamma madoom ho jati hai

c. Raat me nazar nahi aata hai

d. Quwwate lamsa madoom ho jati hai

173. Sikta maigateeta qism hai:

a. Sikta safrawi ki

b. Sikta damwi ki

c. Sikta balghami ki

d. None of the above

174. Zanqa Hurqata muzmina kis marz ko kahte hai:

a. Syphilis

b. Qaroohe masana

c. Iltihabe masana

d. Suzak muzmin

175. Marz epilepsy ka Unani name hai:

a. Qazoon

b. Qassi

c. Aqraba

d. Mazoon

176. Zaroore abaiyaz kis marz me mustamil hai:

a. Ruaaf

b. Rumad

c. Bawaseer

d. Nawaseer

177. Qarha masana ki soorat me boul ke sath kis rang ke Qashoor kharij hote hai:

a. Surkh

b. Surkhi mail

c. Sufaid

d. Sufaidi mail

178. Iltihabe kabid qashbi ki muddat hizant kitni hoti hai:

a. 10 days

b. 15 days

c. 20 days

d. 60-90 days

179. Melancholia ke sath junoon paida hota hai:

a. Ahtaraqe dam se

b. Ahtaraqe safra se

c. Ahtaraqe balgham se

d. Ahtaraqe sauda se

180. Haemophilus pertusis jarasheem kis marz ka sabab hai:

a. Bronchitis

b. Shaheeqa

c. Zeeqan nafas

d. Zatul janab

181. Fasarruddam me koun si dawa mufeed hai:

a. Jawarish jalinoos

b. Jawarish zarooni

c. Dawaus shifa

d. Habbe Izaraqi

182. Nushkha khalal shikam kis Tibbi matab ka hai:

a. Tibbi matab Iraani

b. Tibbi matab Arabi

c. Tibbi matab Lucknowi

d. Tibbi matab Delhi

183. Numla shafooiya ka jai waqooh hota hai:

a. Lip

b. Penis

c. Tongue

d. Head

184. Sibate Irqi darasal wah halat hai:

a. Jis me neend ke sath hizyaan bhi ho

b. Jis me neend ke sath baidari bhi ho

c. Jis me gahri neend hoa karti hai

d. Jis me sirf baidaari hoa karti hai

185. Naume mufrat ka doosra naam:

a. Coma

b. Behoshi

c. Sabat

d. Baidaari

186. Hissate kuliya ki tauleed kis se hoa karti hai:

a. Ajzai ramlia

b. Ajzai nabatia

c. Baroodat se

d. Ghaliz ratoobat se

187. Waram jab nafas dimagh me hota hai to:

a. Nabz azim hone ke baojood mauji hoti hai

b. Azim to hoti hai magar mauji nahi hoti

c. Saree wa mutwatir ho jati hai

d.Sulb wa quwwa ho jati hai

188. Gashi wah marz hai jis me:

a. Tanafus ke sath his wa harkat ki baishtar quwwate muattil ho jati hai

b. Tanafus kesiwa sath his wa harkat ki baishtar quwwate muattil ho jati hai

c. Both

d. Yeh baat marz ki shiddat wa khiffat par munhasar hai

189. Koun si quwwat ka futoor junoon ka sabab banti hai:

a. Quwwate hassasia

b. Quwwate fikaria

c. Quwwate aqalia

d. Quwwate lamisa

190. Marz shifaqaloos ka sabab hoa karta hai:

a. Ghalba wa tafun dam

b. Ghalba wa tafun safra

c. Tafun safra

d. Ghalba dam

191. Wajaul qalb ke daura ke waqt auallan istemaal karna chhaiye:

a. Khameera Gaozaban ambari jawahar wala +Jawahar mohra

b. Dawaul Misk motadil jawahar wala +Jawahar mohra

c. Jawarish zarooni sada +Jawahar mohra

d. Majoon dabeedul warad +Jawahar mohra

192. Sabara kis marz ki qism hai:

a. Sarsam ki

b. Melancholea ki

c. Saraa ki

d. None of the above

193. Humme raba ka ilaj agar na ho sake to is ke khas complication me shamil hai:

a. Zaufe qalb

b. Zaufe meda

c. Istisqa

d. Warme colon

194. Advia zahar mohra wa Tabasheer ka istemaal kis marz me karte hai:

a. Zaufe meda me

b. Zaufe baah me

c. Zaufe kabid me

d. Haiza me

195. Tashanuj matab me badan ka tanqia karte hain:

a. Maaul usool aur iyaraj faiqra se

b. Maul asal se

c. Qai se

d. Fasad se

196. Nafaseul middah kise kahte hai:

a. Dam ka monh ke rah kharij hona

b. Reem ka monh ke rah kharij hona

c. Boul ka kharij hona

d. Baraz kharij hona

197. Marz Ilattul Kubraa Paida hota hai:

a. Damwi madda se

b. Safrawi madda se

c. Saudawi madda se

d. Balghami madda se

198. Mastoqad uffonat se kiya muraad hai:

a. Wah Jarasheem jo uffonat ka baas hote hai

b. Wah akhlat jo uffonat ka baas hote hai

c. Wah kaifiat jo uffonat ka baas hote hai

d. Wah muqaam jaha uffonatt paida hoti hai

199. Babae Tufiliat kise kahte hai:

a. Leewen Hock ko

b. Fransco Redi ko

c. Goege ko

d. Rudolphi ko

200. Kis ghulaf ko Miraaq ke naam se jana jata hai?

a. Pericardium ko

b. Pleura ko

c. Peritoneum ko

d. Perosteum ko

TEST YOUR KNOWLEDGE (MODEL 2)
(AMRAZ-E-NISWAN AND MOALAJAT)
ANSWER KEY

1. B	2. B	3. A	4. D	5. B
6. B	7. C	8. B	9. D	10. A
11. A	12. C	13. B	14. A	15. D
16. B	17. D	18. C	19. A	20. B
21. B	22. D	23. B	24. C	25. C
26. D	27. D	28. D	29. C	30. D
31. A	32. B	33. D	34. C	35. A
36. B	37. C	38. D	39. D	40. B
41. A	42. C	43. D	44. B	45. B
46. C	47. D	48. D	49. A	50. A
51. C	52. B	53. C	54. D	55. D
56. C	57. D	58. D	59. B	60. A
61. D	62. D	63. D	64. C	65. D
66. D	67. A	68. A	69. D	70. D
71. D	72. A	73. C	74. C	75. B
76. A	77. C	78. A	79. D	80. A
81. D	82. D	83. D	84. A	85. A
86. D	87. C	88. D	89. D	90. C
91. A	92. D	93. B	94. C	95. D
96. B	97. C	98. C	99. A	100.C
101.A	102.B	103.D	104.B	105.C
106.C	107.B	108.B	109.D	110.D
111.A	112.C	113.D	114.B	115.A
116.C	117.D	118.D	119.C	120.D
121.C	122.C	123.C	124.D	125.B
126.B	127.B	128.D	129.C	130.D
131.D	132.C	133.A	134.A	135.B
136.C	137.D	138.B	139.A	140.A
141.C	142.C	143.C	144.D	145.A
146.A	147.B	148.C	149.D	150.A

151.D 152.B 153.C 154.D 155.A
156.B 157.C 158.D 159.C 160.B
161.C 162.D 163.B 164.B 165.C
166.D 167.A 168.B 169.C 170.D
171.A 172.B 173.C 174.D 175.A
176.B 177.C 178.D 179.C 180.B
181.C 182.D 183.A 184.B 185.C
186.D 187.A 188.B 189.C 190.A
191.A 192.B 193.C 194.D 195.A
196.B 197.C 198.D 199.D 200.C

TEST YOUR KNOWLEDGE (MODEL 3)
(ADVIA AND KULIYAT)

1. Bazarulkhakham kis ka mutradif naam hai:
a. Saalab mishri
b. Aspaghol
c. Tukhm Rehan
d. Toudri

2. Darhald podhe ka koun sa juz hai:
a. Wood
b. Seeds
c. Post beikh
d. Ushara

3.Saqmonia ki miqdaare khurak hai:
a. 500 mg
b. 3-5 gm
c. 2-4 gm
d. 125-250 mg

4. Shakar Tighals ka mutradif naam hai:
a. Shakar surkh
b. Shakar sufaid
c. Gurh
d. None of the above

5. Sankhia ke istemaal se Qaroorah ka rang tabdeel ho jata hai:
a. Banafshi
b. Surkh
c. Arguawani
d. Siyah

6. Kounch ka podha kaisa hota hai:
a. Bail hoti hai
b. Darakht hai
c. Small podhaha hai
d. Mafroosh booti hai

7. Jalapa ka koun sa juz istemaal hota hai:
a. Shagofa
b. Chhal
c. Beikh
d. Tukhm

8. Dhanab ki istalah kis ke liye mustamil hai:
a. Goudanti
b. Hajarul Yahood
c. Sange jarahat
d. Abrak

9. Warme Tihal me mustamil hai:
a. Barge Kondi sabz
b. Barge Mako sabz
c. Barge Jhao sabz
d. Barge Kasni sabz

10. Piyaz dashti ka nabati naam hai:
a. Urginia indica
b. Cilia indica
c. Allium sativum
d. Aristolochia indica

11. Mako ka nabati naam kiya hai:
a. Solanum tuberosum
b. Solanum nigrum
c. Polygonum bistorta
d. Bresica nigra

12. Ek musafi khoon dawa hai:

a. Bozidan

b. Sina makki

c. Sindooras

d. Suranjan

13. Uslussos ka johare fuaal hai:

a. Glycyrrhmarine

b. Glycyrrhizine

c. Glabsin

d. Phytosterol

14. Morphine ka numayaa fail hai:

a. Analgesic

b. Antipyretics

c. Anti inflammatory

d. Anti emetics

15. Panbadana ka nabati name:

a. Rauwolfia serpentine

b. Gossypium herbaceum

c. Citrus medicus

d. Anacyclus pyratrhum

16. Jadwar ke mawaqae istemaal me shamil hai:

a. Saraa

b. Falij

c. Muqwwi baah

d. Raasha

17. Arosa ka nabati name kiya hai:

a. Acorus calamus

b. Myrtus communis

c. Terminalia arjuna

d. Adhatoda vasica

18. Ajwain khurasani ki mohlik miqdaare khurak:
a. 1 gm
2. More than2 gm
c. More than 5 gm
d. 250 mg

19. Amaltas ke afal:
a. Qabiz, habis
b . Mushil, mudir haiz
c. Muqawwi aasab, dafai bukhar
d. Muqawwi qalb. Mufarreh

20. Dawaushifa me asrol and Mirch siyah ki miqdaar ka tanasub kiya hota hai:
a. 1:1
b. 1:2
c. 1:3
d. 1:4

21. Ahmar ka juze khas hai:
a. Zingar
b. Sange jarahat
c. Sufaida kashgiri
d. Mus sokhta

22. Darchikna murakkab hai:
a. Shangaraf aur raskapoor ka
b. Sankhia aur para ka
c. Fitkari aur para ka
d. None of the above

23. Izaraqi ka mutradif hai:
a. Kuchla
b. Habbul ghurab
c. Qatilul qalb
d. All of the above

24. Habbul rashad ka mutradif name:
a. Haloon
b. Kaknaj
c. Kuchla
d. Jamal gota

25. Chhar tukhm me koun si dawa shamil nahi hai:
a. Tukhm Rehan
b. Tukhm kanocah
c. Tukhm sibat
d. Tukhm aspaghol

26. The shel life of afiyun is:
a. 20 years
b. 10 years
c. 100 years
d. 50 years

27. Arqe ajeeb arq hai:
a. Podina ka
b. Ajwain ka
c. Gaozaban ka
d. None of the above

28. Kushta baizae murgh ki tarkeeb bataiye:
a. Upplo ki aanch de
b. Namkeen paani me ubalein
c. Arqe gulab me 15 din tak tar rakhe
d. Bajar patt ka tareeqa ka istemaal kare

29. Pukhta kushta sammulfar ko shinakht karne ka tareeqa bataie:
a. Paani ki satah par dala jaye to teerta rahe
b. Aag par dala jaye to dhua na de
c. Aag par dalne se rang surkh ho jaye

d. Aag par dalne se rang zarad ho jaye

30. Maghz tukhm kharpaza juze khas hai:
a. Sharbate bazoori motadil
b. Sharbate Dinar
c. Sikanjabeen bazoori
d. Banadaqul bazoori

31. Ehtabase tams ke liye ek mufeed murakkab hai:
a. Jawarish qurtum
b. Ayaraj faiqra
c. Jawarish mastagi
d. Majoon Ushba

32. Wah murakkab jo baah ko barangekhta karta hai:
a. Dawaul misk
b. Majoon kotwali
c. Majoon mubhi antaki
d. Khameera sadaf

33. Qurs malti basant ka mahal istemaal hai:
a. Baraye taqwiyate jigar
b. Baraye taqwiyate aasab
c. Baraye zaheer muzmin
d. Baraye zaheer haad wa tahtul haad

34. Habbe jawahar ki miqdare khurak:
a. 1-2gm goli
b. 5gm goli
c. 2-5 gm goli
d. 1-6 gm goli

35. Resin is dissolved in:
a. water
b. Organic salven
c. Both

d. None

36. Sharbat ke qiwam me shaker ki miqdaar kitni hoti hai:
a. 70%
b. 75%
c. 80%
d. 85%

37. Unani dawa sazi me mutaamila hararat ki taqseem:
a. 4
b. 2
c. 6
d. None

38. Tahmees kea mal se kisi dawa ki:
a. Quwwate amal barh jati hai
b. Quwwate tafteeh barh jati hai
c. Quwwate mushila barh jati hai
d. Quwwate qabiza barh jati hai

39. Firdosul hikmat ka musanif:
a. Buqrat
b. Jalinoos
c. Rhazi
d. Raban Tabri

40. Jo cheez badan me dakhil hoti haim wah asar karti hai:
a. Bilkaifiyat, bil madda, bil joahar
b. Bil kaifiyat
c. Bil madda
d. Bil johar

41. Us dawa ka naam batao jo bairooni aurame sulb ko tahleel karti hai jabki andaroono taur par auram ki salabat me izafa karti hai:

a. Rasoot

b. Kishneez

c. Tisso

d. Zanjabeel

42. Murawaqain kis dawa hai:

a. Warme kabid ki

b. Fracture ki

c. Bawaseer ki

d. Nawaseer ki

43. Baboona murakkabul quwwa dawa hai jis me koun si do quwwate payi jati hai:

a. Tahleel wa jazb

b. Tahleel wa qabz

c. Tahleel wa radaee

d. Tahleel wa taskeen

44. Hasoo kahte hai:

a. Kuskus Shaeer ko

b. Jubn ko

c. Hareera ko

d. Haleeb ko

45. Mufatte hissat dawa hai:

a. jawakhar

b. kalonji

c. Razyana

d. Qaranfal

46. Wah dawa jo lesdaar madda ko kat chant kare:

a. Munjiz

b. Mufajir

c. Murkhi

d. Muqatae

47. Ek muqawwi aazae raisa dawa ki mishal hai:

a. Kajo

b. Sheetraj

c. Ushba

d. Jadwar

48. Murakkabul quwwa dawa ke aqsaam:

a. 4

b. 2

c. 5

d. None

49. Farfiyoon ki shelf life kiya hai:

a. 40 years

b. 50 years

c. 110 years

d. 76 years

50. Kitabul saidna fit Tib ka musanif:

a. Ibne Rushd

b. Ibne Baitaar

c. Albairooni

d. Ibne Sina

51. Tibbim Maqasad ke liye sabse bahtareen Maaul jubn kis janwar ka hota hai:

a. Bakari ka

c. Cow ka

c. Buffalo ka

d. Camel ka

52. Wah Sayyal dawa ji jild ko rangne ke kaam layi jati hai:

a. Tila

b. Zimad

c. Sibagh

d. Khizab

53. Samagh arabi jis darakht se hasil hoti hai us ka naam hai:

a. Andira araroba

b. Amartus cardatus

c. Acrus calomus

d. Acacia Senegal

54. Gale me dawa ki taleeq ka taluque Kis se hai:

a. Soorate nauiya se

b. Roohaniyat se

c. Mizaj

d. Nafsiyat se

55. Dawa sammi ka asar sadir hota hai:

a. Quwwat se

b. Kimiyat se

c. Kaifiat se

d. None of the above

56. Zeera siyah ka mutradif:

a. Zeera kamoni

b. Razyana

c. Bozidaan

d. Hulba

57. Mandarja zail me kiya alkaloid nahi hai:

a. Morphine

b. Digoxin

c. Ajmaline

d. Papaverine

58. Darasal ek dawa doosri dawa ka badal hoti hai:
a. Mushahbiyat ki waja se
b. Colour ki waja se
c. Fail wa tasheer ki bina par
d. Mizaji tazad ki bina par

59. Risalatul Advia wa qalbiabka musanif:
a. Ibne Baitaar
b. Ibne Sina
c. Infaqi
d. Ibne Rushd

60. Sehat mand jigar ke liye muzir lekin warme jigar me mufeed dawa hai:
a. Tukhm kadu
b. Gule Aak
c. Kutki
d. Inzeer

61. Hirrifat-e-salasa is called:
a. Khizab
b. Toodrain
c. Tirkuta
d. Triphal

62. Anupaan is called:
a. Arq of paan
b. Paani
c. Doodh
d. Badreqa

63. Jau Muqashahar is called:

a. Aseer

b. Ghaat

c. Nughda

d. Jawakhar

64. Not included in the chatubeej:

a. Ajwain

b. Kalonji

c. Zeera

d. Halon

65. Farfiyoon is a:

a. Seed

b. Root

c. Flower

d. Latex

66. Darchikna ki kemiyavi ajazae tarkeebi:

a. Arsenic sulphate

b. Arsenic chloride

c. Mercuric sulphate

d. Mercurous chloride

67. Sanbul Teeb ka nabati name:

a. Valertana mallichii

b. Valertana jatamansi

c. Valertana officinalis

d. Valertana album

68. Hyocyamus albus kiya hai:

a. Beesh

b. Ajwain kharasani

c. Ajwain

d. Bachh

69. Mako ke podhe ka nabati name:

a. Solanum indicum

b. Solanum jaguini

c. Solanum lycopersicum

d. Solanum nigrum

70. Reserpine alkaloid ka makhaz hai:

a. Rauwolfia serpintina

b. Strycnous nuxvomica

c. Hyocyamus niger

d. None of the above

71. Uric acid ko kharij karti hai:

a. Asgandh

b. Bozidan

c. Suranjan

d. Kholinjan

72. Ek jigar ke waram ko tahleel karne wali dawa hai:

a. Arqe Gaozaban

b. Arqe baid mushk

c. Arqe baranjasif

d. Arqe ajwain

73. Mohalile awram dawa par nishan lagaye:

a. Afsanteen

b. Ajwain desi

c. Asgandh

d. Uslusoos

74. Aqrab sokhta ki faily taseer hai:

a. Mufattite hissat

b. Mudir boul

c. Mudir haiz

d. Mufatteh hassat

75. Quwwate basarat ko tez karne wali dawa:

a. Doodhi

b. Khardal

c. Ratan jot

d. Dekamali

76. Ziabetus ki ek mufeed dawa hai:

a. Tephrosia purpruea

b. Allium cepa

c. Nardostachys jatamansi

d. Urginia indica

77. Jadwar ki miqdare khurak kiya hai:

a. 2-3 gm

b. 3-5 gm

c. 500 mg-1 gm

d. 100 mg

78. The action of Ghariqoon is:

a. Muqaww-e-bah

b. Mus-hil akhlat-e-salas

c. Mugharri

d. Mufarreh

79. Koun si dawain khali stomach me istemaal karane se meda me kharash paida hoti hai:

a. Antacids and triglycerides

b. Riboflavin

c. Iron salt and salicylates

d. Penicillins

80. Which of following drugs is not a broad spectrum?
a. Penicillins
b. Gentamicin
c. Amoxycillin
d. Tetracycllin

81. Itrifal ke mozid ka naam likhye:
a. Arasto
b. Jalinoos
c. Indaro Makhis
d. Zakaria Rhazi

82. Qairooti kia hai:
a. Shahad aur Zafran ka ameezah
b. Roghan aur Moam ka ameezah
c. Para ke sath koi doosri dhat mili ho
d. Gondhi hoi neem munzamid cheez

83. Afshurda does means:
a. Extract
b. Rind
c. Powder
d. Mucilage

84. Jawarish kamooni ka juze khas:
a. Lemo
b. Zanjabeel
c. Filfil siyah
d. Zeera siyah

85. Who is the inventor of syrup?
a. Buqrat
b. Fesaghorus
c. Jalinoos
d. Ibn-e-Baitar

86. Amraze balghami and saudawi me mufeed murakkab hai:

a. Khameera Sandal

b. Majoon Sakbenj

c. Majoon Seer Alvi khan

d. Majoon Sangdana Murg

87. Qurse Mussalas ka juze khas likhe:

a. Shaheeqa me mufeed hai

b. Shaqeeqa me mufeed hai

c. Wajaul fawad me mufeed hai

d. Qoolinj mirrarah me mufeed hai

88. Munawim dawa ka naam batao:

a. Habbe Shifa

b. Qurse dawaus Shifa

c. Qurs kafoor

d. Qurs Tabasheer

89. Sharbate Ejaz ka ka nafa khas kiya hai:

a. Nafae sual

b. Mussafi khoon

c. Mudir boul

d. Musakine attash hai

90. Jis ka nafa khas taqwiyate jigar hai:

a. Majoon Aqrab

b. Majoon Dabidul warad

c. Majoon Ushba

d. Majoon Najaah

91. Majoon najaah ka nafa khas kkiya hai:

a. Malencholea me mufeed hai

b. Sarsam me mufeed hai

c. Kaboos me mufeed hai

d. Nazla me mufeed hai

92. Barshasha ki miqdare khurak:

a. ½ gm

b. 1 gm

c. 2 gm

c. All of the above

93. The Haleeb is prepared with:

a. Milk

b. Salt

c. Light oil

d. Sugar

94. Pataal Jantar kise kahte hai:

a. Roghan kasheed karne ka aala hai

b. Arq kasheed karne ka aala hai

c. Roghan wa Arq kasheed karne ka aala hai

d. Aala tasyeed hai

95. Kis sayyal cheez ko garam karke jhaag utar kar mail saaf karne kea mal ko istalahan kahte hai:

a. Irgha

b. Ishnaan

c. Ihraaq

d. Taqleem

96. The murakkab useful in visceral inflammation of:

a. Arq Branjasif

b. Itreefal Kishneezi

c. Kustha Musallus

d. Jawarish Bisbasha

97. Kushta banana ke liye Jadeed Aala ka istemaal kiya jata hai is ka naam hai:
a. Pulverizer
b. Mixer grander
c. Refractrometer
d. Muffle furnace

98. Phoolo ka oil nikalne ka tareeqa:
a. Til ke oil me daal kar
b. Eggs ki sufaidi me daal kar
c. Kolho me daal kar
d. All of the above

99. Arand aur mako ke barg ke paani se madder kiya jata hai:
a. Para
b. Afiyun
c. Sammulfar
d. Jamal gota

100. Ek chawal kis ke barabar hota hai:
a. 5.58 mg
b. 4.5 mgc.
c. 3.5 mg
d. 3.8 mg

101. Ratoobate Oola kaha nahi payi jati hai:
a. Shirayaan
b. Avarda
c. Urooqe shaariya
d. Urooqe lympphavia

102. Takabbud se kiya muraad hai:
a. Jiryane khoon
b. Tauleede khoon
c. Taqleele khoon

d. Injamade khoon

103. Alqanoon Fit Tibb ki all five volume ka urdo tarjumah kis ne kiya:
a. Khuwazja Rizwan
b. Allama kabiruddin
c. Allama ghulam hussain Kantoori
d. Hakeem Hadi Hassan

104. Hisse Mustarak ka fail kiya hai:
a. Quwwate muharika wa mudrika ko yakja karna
b. Quwwate Shokia wa Faila ko yakja karna
c. Hawase khamsa ki maloomaat par faisla lena
d. Hawase khamsa batina ko mushtarak karna

105. Koun sa boul Tabai hai?
a. Boule Tabani hai
b. Boule utarji
c. Boule ghusali
d. None of the above

106. Taafun paida karne ke liye ratoobat ke sath aur kiya zaroori hai:
a. Baroodat
b. Yaboosat
c. Hararat
d. None of the above

107. Balgham khoon me kis tarah tabdeel hota hai:
a. Bazariya ihtaraq
b. Bazariya injamad
c. Bazariya nujaz
d. Bazariya tahleel

108. Darje zail me istifraghe kulli kis se hota hai:
a. Qai
b. Fasad

c. Ishal

d. Taareeq

109. Hazam ki akhri manzil kiya hai:
a. Ghiza ka jigar me pahunch jana

b. Jigar me khilt ka banana

c. Khilt ka johare uzu banna

d. Ghair munhazim ghiza ka badan se kharij hona

110. Jitni aqsaam quwwa ki utni hi aqsaam kis ki hain:
a. Akhlat

b. Aaza

c. Mizaj

d. Afaal

111.Abu sahal masihi aur Sahibe kamil ne khoon ko kis se tashbiyah de hai?
a. Water

b. Aabe angoor se

c. Honey se

d. Milk se

112. Koun si quwwat ghiza ko uzue mughtazi ke manind banati hai:
a. Quwwate ghazia

b. Quwwate Namia

c. Quwwate Mugaiyara Oola

d. Quwwate Sammia

113. Rooh ki taareef ka fuzla kis shakal me khariz hota hai:
a. Arq

b. Boul

c. Baraz

d. Dukhaan

114. 23 June se 22 september tak kis fasal ka jamana hai:

a. Fasale saif

b. Fasale khareef

c. Fasale shitaa

d. Fasale rabee

115. Tasauoorat me tarkeeb wa tafseel koun si quwwat karti hai:

a. Quwwate khyyal

b. Hisse mustarak

c. Quwwate Wahima

d. Quwwate mutsarifa

116. Kis quwwat ke munqata hone se uzue mutaaffin wa fasid ho jata hai:

a. Quwwate Haiwania

b. Quwwate Nafsania

c. Quwwate Tabiyah

d Quwwate Tanasulia

117. Darje zail me Ibne Haisham ki kitab koun si hai:

a. Kitabul Taiseer

b. Kitabul Tasreef

c. Kitabul Manazir

d. Taqweemul sahta

118. Khoon me makhloot hone ke alawah safra ka insabab kha hoti hai:

a. Lungs

b. Potahepatis

c. Doudenum

d. Jigar

119. Aota qalb ki kiya khidmat anzam deta hai:

a. Khidmate muhayya

b. Khidmate muaddiya

c. Khidmate injazab

d. Khidmate inhazam

120. Mizaj motadil Tibbi ki qisme:

a. 4

b. 8

c. 12

d. 16

121. Aqleem kitne hain:

a. 3

b. 4

c. 5

d. 7

122. Moaleed kitne hain:

a. 2

b. 3

c. 4

d. 5

123. Aazae mufrada ki aqsaam kitni hain:

a. 5

b. 6

c. 7

d. 10

124. Safra ghair tabai kitne qism ka hota hain:

a. 2

b. 3

c. 4

d. 5

125. Aamaar (Ages) kitne hain:

a. 3

b. 4

c. 5
d. 6

126. Uzn ke kitne hisse hain:
a. 2
b. 3
c. 4
d. 5

127. Quwwai Tabaiya khadima kitne hain:
a. 2
b. 3
c. 4
d. 5

128. Quwwate ghazia kitne quwwa par mustaamil hoti hai:
a. 3
b. 4
c. 5
d. 7

129. Khoon ka mizaj hota hai:
a. Har ratab
b. Barid ratab
c. Har yabis
d. Barid yabis

130. Asbabe Waja kitne hai:
a. 2
b. 3
c. 4
d. 5

131. Alamate amzaja kitne hain?
a. 5

b. 6
c. 8
d. 10

132. Zafrani (Ahmar naasai) rang ka qaroora kis kaifiat marzi par dalalat karta hai:

a. Shadeed yaboosat par dalalat karta hai
b. Shadeed baroodat par dalalat karta hai
c. Humme muhariqa par dalalat karta hai
d. Humme moaziba par dalalat karta hai

133. Boule ghusali kis marz par dalalat karta hai:

a. Amraze meda par
b. Amraze riya par
c. Amraze jigar wa amraze gurda par
d. Amraze aama par

134. Fussol kitne hai:

a. 2
b. 3
c. 4
d. 5

135. Jalinoos ke according ahwale badan kitne hain:

a. 3
b. 4
c. 5
d. 6

136. Badtareen mausam koun sa hai:

a. Mausam saif badtareen mausam hai
b. Mausam khareef badtareen mausam hai
c. Mausamrabee badtareen mausam hai
d. Mausam shitaa badtareen mausam hai

137. Asbabe mubarida kitne qism ke hain:

a. 2

b. 3

c. 4

d. 5

138. Asbabe musakhina kitne qism ke hain:

a. 2

b. 3

c. 4

d. 5

139. Normal count of WBC:

a. 2000-6000/cm

b. 4000-11000/cm

c. 8000-15000/cm

d. 1000-25000/cm

140. Iltihaab and indimaal me aham role hai:

a. Kurriyate hamara

b. Kurriyate baize ka

c. Kurriyate damawia ka

d. None of the above

141. Azla kis tarkeeb se murakkab hai:

a. Tarkeebe awwal

b. Tarkeebe sani

c. Tarkeebe salisa

d. Tarkeebe rabai

142. Boule ahmar ki aqsaam hain:

a. wardi, nari, ahmarqaani

b. ashab, ashqar, zafrani

c. wardi, ahmarqaani. Ashab

d. Nari, ahmar qaani, ashab

143. Ajnase nabz ki tadaad hai:

a. 4

b. 6

c. 8

d. 10

144. Mazah ke lihaz se ghair tabai balgham ki aqsaam hain:

a. malah, zujazi, affis

b. Hamiz, affis, jussi

c. Malah, hamiz, affis

d. Affis, zujazi, hamiz

145. Azae barida ki tarteeb hai:

a. Asaab, ghazroof, rabat , haddi

b. haddi, ghazroof,rabat , asaab

c. haddi, rabat, Assab, ghazroof

d.Ghazroof ,haddi, assab, rabat

146. Ibne Sina ke lihaz se nabz ki harkat hai:

a. Harkate kaifia

b. Harkate ainia

c. Harkate kinia

d. Harkate wazaia

147. Majari ke tang hone ka sabab ho sakta hai:

a. Shiddat baroodat

b. Quwwate masika ka zauf hona

c.Advia mushila ka istemaal

d. Advia murkhia ka istemaal

148. Khalis warmw damvi ko kahte hai:

a. Warme humrah

b. Warme humarah falghamooni

c. Warme fakghamooni

d. Warme falghamooni humarah

149. Amraze rabee me shumar hota hai:
a. Ruaf, ishale damwi, wa khunaaq ka
b. Humme ghib, busoore safaravi. Wa asoobe chasm ka
c. Jurb, qooba, usrul boul
d. Sartan , arqunnisa, hikka

150. Fataq tafarruqe ittesal hai:
a. Azla ka
b. Shirayain
c. Aghshiah ka
d. Asaab ka

151. Arq kis hazam ka fuzla hai:
a. Hazne medi
b. Hazne kabdi
c. Hazne urooqi
d. Hazne uzwi

152. Matraqi, sindani and rakabi kis fail me maaun hain:
a. Faile samaa
b. Faile injazab
c. Faile basar
d. Faile inkabab

153. Nabz zanbul far kis shakal ki hoti hai:
a. Daira numa
b. Murabba numa
c. M akhrooti numa
d. None of the above

154. Dalak ka shumar kis asbab me hota hai:
a. Asbabe zarooriya
b. Asbabe maddiya
c. Asbabe ghair zarooriya

d. Asbabe tammamia

155. Afyun kis quwwat ko quwwa karti hai:
a. Quwwate jazba ko
b. Quwwate hazma ko
c. Quwwate masika ko
d. Quwwate dafia ko

156. Marze adad kis me shamil hai:
a. Ajnashe ushra me
b. Sue mizaj
c. Sue tarkeeb
d. Tafarruqe ittesal

157. Lafz baseet kis se mansoob hai:
a. Tabiyat
b. Arkan
c. Akhlat
d. Quwwa

158. Harkat ka mizaj kiya hai:
a. Har
b. Barid
c. Ratab
d. None of the above

159. Halate badan me Taqabil tazad ka nazariya kis ne paish kiya:
a. Buqrat
b. Jalinoos
c. Ibne zakaria Rhaze
d. Ibne Sina

160. Nabz azim saree mutfawit kis halat me milti hai:
a. Naum ki halat me
b. Harkat ki halat me

c. Ghussa ki halat me
d. Dard ki halat me

161.Quwwate shoqia kis ka hissa hai:
a. Quwwate muhasila
b. Quwwate muharika
c. Quwwate tanasulia
d. Quwwate wahima

162. Quwwate masika kaha payi jati hai:
a. Meda me
b. Jigar me
c. Aama me
d. Har uzu me

163. Saikhur rais ke mutabique ahwale badan kahte hai:
a. 1
b. 2
c. 3
d. 4

164. Sabab johri kiya hai:
a. hararat
b. Baroodat
c. Ghum wa ghussa
d. Ghiza

165. Asbabe badaniya me kiya shamil nahi hai:
a. Asbabe khiltia
b. Asbabe mizajia
c. Asbabe ghizaia
d. Asbabe takeebia

166. Istiwa wa ikhtilaf ka shumaar kis me hota hai:
a. Maqoolate ushra

b. Ajnasebushra

c. Adilla nabz

d. Adilla baraz

167. Balgham Tabai ki khas sifat kiya hai:

a. Ba asani tahleel ho jana

b. Ba asani nuzaj pa jana

c. Ba asani jism se kharij ho jana

d. Ba asani khoon me ho jana

168. Zakheera khuarzam Shahi ka urdu tarjuma kis ne kiya:

a. Dr Ghulam Jeelani

b. Hakeem kabiruddin

c. Hakeem Nayyar Wasti

d. Hakeem Hadi Hassan

169. Dauraane khoom ko saree karne me maaoon koun hai:

a. Naum

b. Sukoon

c. Harkat

d. Tarweeh

170. Uffonat ke liyy koun se kaifiat sazgar mahoul paida karti hai:

a. Sard khushk

b. Sard wa tar

c. Garam khushk

d. Garam wa tar

171. Asbabe zarooriya me koun sa sabab shamil nahi hai?

a. Hawa

b. Maqool wa Mashroob

c. Harkat wa sukoone badani

d. Ghusl wa hammam

172. Shaikhurrais abu ali Sina ke nazdeek aqleem ziyadah motadil hai:
a. Aqleem awwal khate istiwa ke qareeb
b. Aqleem dom
c. Aqleem soom
d. Aqleem chharum

173. Quwwate wahima ka shumar kis me hota hai:
a. Quwwate Tabiyah me
b. Hawase zahira me
c. Hawse batina me
d. Quwwate khayal me

174. Jumla ratoobat badan bunyaddi taur par kitne Guroho me me taqseem hain:
a. 2
b. 4
c. 6
d. 8

175. Sauda ghair Tabai ki kitni qisme hai:
a. 2
b. 4
c. 6
d. 8

176. Mirrara jigar ke liya kaisa uzu hai:
a. Khadim mubhi
b. Khadim moadi
c. Uzu muqwwi
d. Uzu muzaf

177. Maddah rooh kin ashiya par mustamil hai:
a. Aghzia lateefa

b. Akhlate lateefa

c. Khoon shiryani balgham

d. Khoon vareedi wa safra

178. Manae uffonat koun se khilt hai:
a. Khilte dam

b. Khilte balgham

c. Khilte safra

d. Khilte sauda

179. Koun si khilt har yabis hoti hai:
a. Khlte dam

b. Khlte balgham

c. Khlte safra

d. Khlte sauda

180. Sehat wa marz kin asbab me qaim hote hai:
a. Asbabe maddiya

b. Asbabe faila

c. Asbabe sooria

d. Asbabe tammamia

181. Warm e haad me koun si nabz payi jati hai:
a. Zanbulfaar

b. Matraqi

c. Doodi

d. Minshari

182. Firdousul hikmat likhi hai:
a. Ibne sina

b. Zakaria rhaze

c. Abusahal Masihi

d. None of the above

183. Hazme kabdi ka fuzla hai:
a. Boul

b. Baraz

c. Paseena
d. Safra

184. Safra ke sath raqeeq balgham ki ameezash ko kahte hai:
a. Safra kurrasi
b. Safra muhyya
c. Safra muhyya wa kurrasi
d. Safra mirra

185. Kitabul mansoori fittib likhi hai:
a. Ibne Sina
b. Abubakar Mohammad bin Zakaria Razhe
c. Abul Qasim Zohrawi
d. None of the above

186. Hair bakasrat se ugte hain:
a. Baroodat ki mauzoodgi me
b. Hararat ki mauzoodgi me
b. Hararat wa yaboosat ki mauzoodgi me
d. None of the above

187. Quwwat ke wajood ka sabot kiya hai:
a. Unsur
b. Khilt
c. Usfar
d. Fail

188. Azame matraqi, sindaani and rakabi kis quwwat ke Mauoon hain:
a. Shamma
b.Basira
c. Samia
d. Lamsa

189. Agar do ya do se ziyadah anasir ke milne se in sabikae khawas badal jaye to yeh koun sa mizaj hoga:
a. Mizaje shakhsi
b. Mizaje naui
c. Imtizaje sad
d. Imtizaje haqeeqi

190. Aauia rooh me kiya shamil nahi hai:
a. Shirayin
b. Avarda
c. Urooqe shariya
d. Qasbaturriya

191. Quwwate ghazia ke tahat darje zail koun si quwwat shamil nahi hai:
a. Quwatte dafia
b. Quwatte jaziba
c. Quwatte masika
d. Quwatte Saamia

192. Azae yabisa me shamil hain:
a. Hairs, bones, ligament and cartilage
b. Hairs, nerve, cartilage and brain
c. Bone , cartilage and qalb
d. Sameen Riwaj , nerves and ligaments

193. Dalak istedaad karte hain:
a. Before Hammam
b. Before exercise
c. After exercise
d. None of the above

194. Sufaid rasoob dalat karta hai:
a. Amraze gurda me
b. Amraze masana me
c. Amraze kuliya me

d. Amraze jigar me

195. Qaroora me rasoob ki miqdaar ziyadah hogi:
a. Mosame saif me
b. Mosame shitaa me
c. Mosame khareef me
d. Mosame rabee me

196. Taraveeh se muraad hai:
a. Rooh me garmi paida karna
b. Rooh ke garam mizaj ko etadal par lana
c. Rooh me baroodat paida karna
d. Rooh me tezi paida karna

197. Iltihaab mishal hai:
a. Warme barid ki
b. Warme haar ki
c. Both
d. None

198. Khilt ko uzu ka badal matahalul banana me koun si quwwat hissa leti hai:
a. Quwwate namia
b. Quwatte ghazia
c. Quwwate mughaiyara Oola
d. None of the above

199. Kis umr me insaan ka mizaj motadil tareen hota hai:
a. Sine shaikhokhat
b. Sine kahoolat
c. Sine shabab
d. Sine namu

200. Harate gharizia kis ke ehtaraq se paida hoti hai:
a. Rooh aur balgham ke ehtaraq se
b. Rooh aurdam ke makhsoos ajza ke ehtaraq se

c. Rooh aur safra ke ehtaraq se
d. Rooh aur sauda ke ehtaraq se

TEST YOUR KNOWLEDGE (MODEL 3)
(ADVIA AND KULIYAT)
ANSWERS KEY

1. D	2. A	3. A	4. D	5. D
6. A	7. C	8. D	9. C	10. A
11. B	12. B	13. A	14. A	15. B
16. C	17. D	18. D	19. B	20. A
21. A	22. B	23. D	24. A	25. C
26. D	27. B	28. A	29. B	30. D
31. A	32. B	33. C	34. A	35. B
36. A	37. A	38. D	39. D	40. A
41. B	42. A	43. B	44. C	45. A
46. C	47. D	48. B	49. A	50. C
51. A	52. C	53. D	54. A	55. C
56. A	57. B	58. C	59. B	60. D
61. C	62. D	63. B	64. C	65. D
66. D	67. B	68. B	69. D	70. A
71. C	72. C	73. A	74. A	75. C
76. C	77. C	78. B	79. C	80. B
81. C	82. B	83. A	84. D	85. B
86. C	87. B	88. B	89. A	90. B
91. A	92. D	93. C	94. A	95. A
96. A	97. D	98. A	99. A	100.A
101.D	102.D	103.C	104.C	105.B
106.C	107.C	108.B	109.C	110.D
111.D	112.A	113.D	114.B	115.D
116.A	117.C	118.C	119.B	120.B
121.D	122.B	123.D	124.C	125.B
126.B	127.C	128.A	129.A	130.A
131.D	132.C	133.C	134.C	135.A
136.B	137.D	138.D	139.B	140.B
141.A	142.C	143.D	144.C	145.C
146.D	147.A	148.C	149.A	150.C
151.D	152.A	153.C	154.C	155.C
156.C	157.B	158.A	159.B	160.D

161.B 162.D 163.B 164.D 165.C
166.C 167.D 168.D 169.C 170.D
171.D 172.A 173.C 174.B 175.B
176.B 177.B 178.C 179.C 180.A
181.D 182.D 183.A 184.D 185.B
186.C 187.D 188.C 189.D 190.D
191.D 192.A 193.B 194.B 195.A
196.B   197.B 198.B 199.C 200.B

www.ingramcontent.com/pod-product-compliance
Lightning Source LLC
Chambersburg PA
CBHW051622170526
45167CB00001B/24